REHABILITATION IN
PARKINSON'S DISEASE

FORTHCOMING TITLES

Exercise Physiology for Health Professionals
Stephen Bird

Effective Communication for Health Professionals
Philip Burnard

Occupational Therapy for the Brain-Injured Adult
Jo Clark-Wilson and Gordon Muir Giles

Visual Impairment: Perspectives in practice
Jane Hutchinson

Assessment in Occupational Therapy
Greg Kelly

Early Identification of Language Impairment in Children
James Law

Therapy for the Burn Patient
Annette Leveridge

Speech and Language Problems in Children
Dilys A. Treharne

THERAPY IN PRACTICE SERIES

Edited by Jo Campling

This series of books is aimed at 'therapists' concerned with rehabilitation in a very broad sense. The intended audience particularly includes occupational therapists, physiotherapists and speech therapists, but many titles will also be of interest to nurses, psychologists, medical staff, social workers, teachers or volunteer workers. Some volumes are interdisciplinary, others are aimed at one particular profession. All titles will be comprehensive but concise, and practical but with due reference to relevant theory and evidence. They are not research monographs but focus on professional practice, and will be of value to both students and qualified personnel.

1. Occupation Therapy for Children with Disabilities
   Dorothy E. Penso
2. Living Skills for Mentally Handicapped People
   Christine Peck and Chia Swee Hong
3. Rehabilitation of the Older Patient
   Edited by Amanda J. Squires
4. Physiotherapy and the Elderly Patient
   Paul Wagstaff and Davis Coakley
5. Rehabilitation of the Severely Brain-Injured Adult
   Edited by Ian Fussey and Gordon Muir Giles
6. Communication Problems in Elderly People
   Rosemary Gravell
7. Occupational Therapy Practice in Psychiatry
   Linda Finlay
8. Working with Bilingual Language Disability
   Edited by Deirdre M. Duncan
9. Counselling Skills for Health Professionals
   Philip Burnard
10. Teaching Interpersonal Skills
    A handbook of experiential learning for health professionals
    Philip Burnard
11. Occupational Therapy for Stroke Rehabilitation
    Simon B. N. Thompson and Maryanne Morgan
12. Assessing Physically Disabled People at Home
    Kathy Maczka
13. Acute Head Injury
    Practical management in rehabilitation
    Ruth Garner
14. Practical Physiotherapy with Older People
    Lucinda Smyth et al.

15. Keyboard, Graphic and Handwriting Skills
Helping people with motor disabilities
Dorothy E. Penso

16. Community Occupational Therapy with Mentally Handicapped
Adults
Debbie Isaac

17. Autism
Professional perspectives and practice
Edited by Kathryn Ellis

18. Multiple Sclerosis
Approaches to management
Edited by Lorraine De Souza

19. Occupational Therapy in Rheumatology
An holistic approach
Lynne Sandles

20. Breakdown of Speech
Causes and remediation
Nancy R. Milloy

21. Coping with Stress in the Health Professions
A practical guide
Philip Burnard

22. Speech and Communication Problems in Psychiatry
Rosemary Gravell and Jenny France

23. Limb Amputation
From aetiology to rehabilitation
Rosalind Ham and Leonard Cotton

24. Management in Occupational Therapy
Zielfa B. Maslin

25. Rehabilitation in Parkinson's Disease
Francis I. Caird

Rehabilitation in Parkinson's Disease

Edited by
FRANCIS I. CAIRD DM, FRCP

David Cargill Professor of Geriatric Medicine
University of Glasgow

CHAPMAN & HALL
London · New York · Tokyo · Melbourne · Madras

UK	Chapman & Hall, 2–6 Boundary Row, London SE1 8HN
USA	Chapman & Hall, 29 West 35th Street, New York NY10001
Japan	Chapman & Hall Japan, Thomson Publishing Japan, Hirakawacho Nemoto Building, 7F, 1–7–11 Hirakawa-cho, Chiyoda-ku, Tokyo 102
Australia	Chapman & Hall Australia, Thomas Nelson Australia, 102 Dodds Street, South Melbourne, Victoria 3205
India	Chapman & Hall India, R. Seshadri, 32 Second Main Road, CIT East, Madras 600 035

First edition 1991

© 1991 Francis I. Caird

Phototypeset in Times 10/12 by Input Typesetting Ltd, London
Printed in Great Britain by St Edmundsbury Press Ltd,
Bury St Edmunds, Suffolk

ISBN 0 412 34600 1

British Library Cataloguing in Publication Data
Rehabilitation in Parkinson's disease.
  1. Man. Parkinsons's disease
  I. Caird, F. I. (Francis Irvine)
  616.833

  ISBN 0–412–34600–1

Library of Congress Cataloging-in-Publication Data
Rehabilitation in Parkinson's disease / edited by Francis I. Caird.
      p.   cm.—(Therapy in practice series; 25)
    Includes bibliographical references and index.
    ISBN 0-412-34600-1 (pbk.)
    1. Parkinsonism—Patients—Rehabilitation. 2. Parkinsonism—
Treatment. I. Caird, F. I. (Francis Irvine) II. Series.
    [DNLM: 1. Parkinson Disease—rehabilitation. WL 359 R345]
  RC382.R44 1991
  616.8′3303—dc20
  DNLM/DLC
  for Library of Congress   91-10916 CIP

Contents

Contributors   viii

Preface   ix

1 Parkinson's disease and its natural history   1
  Francis I. Caird

2 Drug therapy of Parkinson's disease   8
  Brian Pentland

3 Nursing care   25
  Barbara K. Sharp

4 Physiotherapy   45
  Moira A. Banks

5 Occupational therapy   66
  Alison Beattie

6 Speech therapy   87
  Sheila Scott

7 The social worker   107
  Mary Baker and Pauline Smith

8 The Parkinson's Disease Society   120
  Mary Baker and Bridget McCall

Useful addresses   128

Index   131

Contributors

Mary Baker, BA, AIMSW
Welfare Director,
Parkinson's Disease Society, London

Moira A. Banks, BA, MCSP
Lecturer in Physiotherapy,
The Queen's College, Glasgow

Alison Beattie, DIPCOT
Research Occupational Therapist,
Southern General Hospital, Glasgow

Francis I. Caird, DM, FRCP
David Cargill Professor of Geriatric Medicine,
University of Glasgow

Bridget McCall, BA (HONS)
Personal Assistant to Welfare Director,
Parkinson's Disease Society

Brian Pentland, BSC, MB, FRCP
Senior Lecturer in Rehabilitation Medicine
University of Edinburgh, and Consultant Physician, Astley
Ainslie Hospital, Edinburgh

Sheila Scott, BSC, MCST
Formerly Research Speech Therapist,
Department of Geriatric Medicine, University of Glasgow

Barbara K. Sharp, RGN, RCSN, RCNT
Formerly lecturer in Nursing Studies,
Department of Nursing Studies, University of Glasgow

Pauline Smith, BSC (HONS)
Education and Training Officer
Parkinson's Disease Society

Preface

Parkinson's disease is a common condition with major and multiple effects both on sufferers and their families and carers. The revolution in its drug therapy in the last twenty years has greatly improved the quality of life of many patients, but the passage of time means that more and more are left with substantial disability. This book attempts to convey the value of a team effort to reduce this and help overcome their difficulties. It must be realized that, although doctors are very important by virtue of their control of drug therapy, others are equally, or on occasions more important to the patient. Any plan of management must be flexible so as to be able to take into account both the vagaries of the disease in the individual patient and all the complex consequences of long-term treatment. Not unnaturally, this book is based on experience in the United Kingdom, where there is detailed knowledge of the crucial role of each of the members of the rehabilitation teams so often deployed there. It attempts to deal with principles and with day-to-day practice rather than with the ever-increasing details of neuroscience in Parkinson's disease. It is intended for nurses and paramedical therapists more than for doctors, but it is to be hoped that they, as members of the team, will also benefit from what is to be found here.

To avoid accusations of sexism, the patient will be referred to throughout as 'he' and 'him', and the nurse and therapist as 'she' and 'her', whatever the truth of the matter.

Our acknowledgements are due to our patients with Parkinson's disease, in particular to members of the Glasgow and West of Scotland branch of the Parkinson's Disease Society, and to its national Welfare Advisory Panel; to Mrs Lesley Manson and Mrs Barbara Haw, Occupational Therapists; and personally to colleagues who have stimulated and maintained my interest in the disease, especially Professor G.A. Broe and Dr W.J. Mutch. The physiotherapeutic exercises in Chapter 4 were drawn from *Living with Parkinson's Disease*, published by the Society. Thanks are also due to the Audiovisual Department of the Southern General Hospital, Glasgow.

F.I.C.

March 1991

1

Parkinson's disease and its natural history

Francis I. Caird

Parkinsonism is a clinical syndrome characterized by four cardinal features: tremor of a particular type, muscular rigidity, slowness and poverty of movement (bradykinesia or hypokinesia), and postural instability. It has several causes (Table 1.1), only two of which are common by themselves, the idiopathic variety (Parkinson's disease, PD), and drug-induced parkinsonism (DIP), whose reported frequency is variable, but may account for as many as half of newly diagnosed cases in elderly hospital patients (Stephen and Williamson, 1984). However, the rarer causes taken together account for a not inconsiderable proportion of cases.

Table 1.1 Parkinsonism and Parkinson's disease

Parkinsonism:

    Idiopathic (Parkinson's disease)

    Drug-induced (especially phenothiazines and butyrophenones)

    Post-encephalitic

    MTP toxicity

Parkinsonism plus:

    Progressive supranuclear palsy (Steele–Richardson syndrome)

    Multiple system atrophy:
       olivopontocerebellar atrophy
       strionigral degeneration
       progressive autonomic failure (Shy–Drager syndrome)

In addition Parkinsonian features can occur in:

    Alzheimer's disease

    Multiple cerebral infarcts

    Head injury (e.g. boxers)

Figure 1.1 Age and prevalence of PD (Mutch *et al.*, 1986)

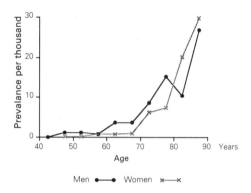

Men ●——● Women ✗┈┈┈✗

PD is one of the commoner neurological diseases. Its prevalence increases with age, so that, according to the most recent reported figures, from approximately one per 1000 under the age of 60 to five per 1000 at the age of 70, and 20 per 1000 over the age of 85 (Mutch *et al.*, 1986; Figure 1.1). At any one time two-thirds of all patients are aged 70 or over. It appears to be equally common the world over, the age-related pattern of prevalence being similar in five continents. The median age at onset in most recent series of patients is in the late 60s, and like its prevalence, the incidence (the number of new cases in unit time) increases with age, but one in seven is diagnosed under the age of 50. Males are slightly more often affected than females, but the sex incidence of PD is, for practical purposes, equal. There is little or no obvious hereditary tendency.

The overall pattern of the epidemiology of PD thus gives little clue as to where to look for a likely cause, since there are neither genetic nor environmental influences (with one exception) of any definite importance. The exception is that cigarette smoking appears to protect against the development of the disease, but clearly this can have no practical importance in prevention, since the price of prevention of PD, in terms of the many and fatal tobacco-related diseases caused, would be unacceptably high. One recent theory suggests the importance of a widespread neurotoxin, which acts in a similar way to MPTP, a by-product of illegal 'drug designing', which produces a rapidly developing Parkinsonian syndrome in both man and animals.

Figure 1.2 Lewy body in neurone in substantia nigra (courtesy of Professor. D.I. Graham)

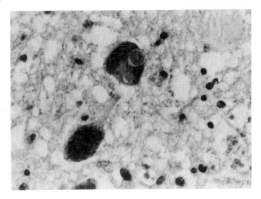

PATHOLOGY

Idiopathic PD is characterized pathologically by degeneration of neurones in the substantia nigra, where the characteristic Lewy bodies (Figure 1.2) are seen in the remaining cells and also in some cases elsewhere in the brain. What they signify is unknown. The cells in question are neurones utilizing dopamine as their transmitter, projecting to the caudate nucleus on the same side of the brain, and concerned essentially with the control of movement. It is on replacement of the lost cerebral dopamine that treatment of PD now largely rests. Eighty per cent or more of cerebral dopamine has to be lost before Parkinsonian symptoms develop, and the condition's relation to age could well be due to the fact that both the dopamine concentration and the number of cells in the substantia nigra that produce it, fall steadily from birth, some 60% or so having been lost in extreme old age. Clearly, the older the person, the smaller the additional deficit in cerebral dopamine, produced by whatever mechanism, that is required to produce Parkinsonian symptoms.

CLINICAL FEATURES

The four primary features of PD, mentioned above, produce clinical symptoms that are numerous and varied. All are relatively inconspicuous at the onset of the disease, so that it is not

3

surprising that diagnosis is frequently delayed by up to several years. Patients and their relatives may complain of this fact, but it is very rare that anything significant has been lost by the delay.

The first symptom is most often tremor of one hand, which later spreads to the other hand and then more widely throughout the body. The tremor is characteristically at a frequency of about five per second; when, as it often does, it involves the thumb, it produces so-called pill-rolling. In the elderly, tremor is less prominent and is often initially variable so requiring prolonged or several periods of observation before it is seen. The tremor is at its maximum when the patient is at rest, tends to improve with movement, is increased by emotion and abolished by sleep.

The limbs are characteristically rigid, their resistance to movement being approximately the same throughout the whole range of movement (lead-pipe rigidity). In the wrist and elbow the rigidity may have a cogwheel feel to it, the phenomenon being due to rigidity interrupted by tremor.

In general bradykinesia and hypokinesia affect the same muscles as tremor and rigidity. It may be seen as difficulty in initiating movement, and particularly rapid alternating movements such as alternating flexion and extension of the fingers as when one plays the piano. One of the most characteristic early symptoms is slowness and awkwardness in turning in bed, and in rising from lying to sitting, and from sitting to standing.

The stance is characteristically flexed at the neck, hips, and knees. The face is immobile, and the normal rate of blinking is much reduced. Bradykinesia particularly affects gait; the patient finds it hard to start walking, and may appear to be glued to the ground. Walking proceeds with small steps, and without any arm swing. Turning is especially a problem, because it is in effect a series of new movements requiring initiation. The patient may be unable to stop walking, and may begin to run uncontrollably (festination). A small proportion have particular difficulty in passing between two pieces of furniture or through a doorway, and may hesitate or stop at these places.

Postural instability impairs the righting reflexes and produces a tendency to fall, so that when the patient sits with his feet off the floor and his hands on his knees, and is pushed to one side, he makes no movement to preserve his posture and save himself (sometimes called the Russian Doll phenomenon). When the patient is standing, gentle pressure over the sternum can start an uncorrectable backwards walking movement.

4

The eye movements are normal. Emotional movement of the face may be particularly impaired. The unresponsive facial appearance combined with the flexed posture of the neck and the general poverty of movement gives rise to the so-called reptilian appearance. It has recently been shown that these features lead health professionals (let alone lay people) to consider those with PD unfeeling, cold, and unattractive when, of course, they are none of these things (Pentland *et al.*, 1987).

Changes in speech may make a substantial proportion of patients (up to half, usually the moderately or severely physically affected) extremely difficult to understand. Speech comes in irregular bursts with prolonged pauses and frequent periods of acceleration. Speech is flat and lacks those changes in pitch and tone which are important in communication, to some extent semantically, and even more because they convey much of the emotional content of spoken speech. A more detailed account is given in Chapter 6. Patients with advanced disease may have very considerable difficulty in swallowing; all phases are affected (see p. 98).

In the early stages of the disease mental function is normal but as many as a third of patients are depressed. However, in the later stages visual hallucinations, which are usually drug-related, and frank dementia, all too often develop.

Other symptoms include increased salivation, leading to embarrassing drooling, and oily skin (seborrhoea).

The functional performance of patients with PD may show remarkable fluctuations throughout the day or from one day to another. Factors such as stress, depression, and cold can affect their motor performance. Many patients suffer from a phenomenon known as 'freezing'. This describes episodes which occur without warning when the patient is unable to complete a motor activity, such as walking, writing, or speaking, and is as if they are frozen. These last for a variable length of time but usually for a few minutes. Patients taking levodopa may experience a particularly unpleasant fluctuation known as 'the on–off phenomenon', aptly named since some liken it to a light being switched on and off: 'off' being the period when there is no response to drugs and the patient is very hypokinetic, and 'on' being the period when the drugs are effective. Some are able to predict when an 'off' period is likely but others have no warning. In these patients it is totally unpredictable. The length of 'off' periods can vary from minutes to hours. Not unnaturally, onlookers (carers, nurses and others) may attribute these periods to 'not trying', with much consequent ill-feeling on both sides.

There are as yet no specific and commonly available investigations or tests for PD, and its diagnosis therefore depends on recognition of its characteristic features, or on demonstration that other features thought to be Parkinsonian are not truly so. Thus for instance, senile or essential tremor is one of the most important differential diagnoses, because this often hereditary condition is as common as PD and is also age-related. In essential tremor, however, the jaw and head are particularly affected; the tremor is slightly less rapid, and is not accompanied by any of the other features of Parkinson's disease, in particular rigidity and bradykinesia. There is rarely any disability.

Untreated, PD progresses slowly over a period of many years. At present and with treatment, this progress is usually halted for as long as five to seven years, but after this time increasing disability, much of it due to other age-related disease, and also progressive difficulties with treatment tend to predominate (Chapter 2), together with psychiatric abnormalities, in particular dementia. Whether dementia is due to PD itself, to other concomitant disease processes (e.g. Alzheimer's disease) or to treatment, is at present not entirely clear, but the last possibility is much the least likely.

In summary, PD is a common condition, giving rise to substantial disability and having both positive (e.g. tremor) and negative features (e.g. bradykinesia), the former being substantially less important than the latter in determining disability.

A POSSIBLE OVERALL STRATEGY FOR THE MANAGEMENT OF PARKINSON'S DISEASE

Consideration of the natural history of Parkinson's disease, and the diagnostic difficulties outlined above suggests that a plan along the following lines for its overall management should be considered. When the diagnosis is suspected, because there is sufficient diagnostic difficulty in a high enough proportion of cases, the patient should be referred to a hospital consultant (neurologist, geriatrician, or general physician) for confirmation of the diagnosis. At this time, consideration should be given to further referral of the patient to one or more of the paramedical therapists for assessment, depending on his particular problems.

This will enable planning of their assistance in the management of the disease from the earliest appropriate moment.

Recommendations should then be made about drug treatment, and the patient can be returned to the care of his general practitioner until any problems arise. The patient should then be referred back to hospital for the necessary expert advice. At this point, maybe three to five years or more into the disease, he should be referred again to the appropriate paramedical therapists. It should then be made possible that, whenever further disability occurs, he should be seen by one or more of them. They would be able to plan for the patient's management, perhaps becoming serially more and more involved as time goes on.

As much therapy as possible should be conducted in the patient's home. This gives all the therapists the opportunity to assess the patient in a real life environment and enables much closer cooperation with partners, relatives, and carers, so as to ensure more effective ongoing therapy.

REFERENCES

Mutch, W.J., Dingwall-Fordyce, I., Downie, A.W., Paterson, J.G. and Roy, S.K. (1986) Parkinson's disease in a Scottish city. *British Medical Journal*, **292**, 534.

Pentland, B., Pitcairn, T.K., Gray, J.M., Riddle, W.J.R. (1987) The effects of reduced expression in Parkinson's disease on impression formation by health professionals. *Clinical Rehabilitation*, **1**, 307.

Stephen, P.J. and Williamson, J. (1984) Drug-induced Parkinsonism in the elderly. *Lancet*, **ii**, 1082.

2

Drug therapy of Parkinson's disease

Brian Pentland

The only treatment suggested by James Parkinson in his original account of the condition which now bears his name, was taking blood from the patient's neck; he felt that until more was known about the cause, internal medicines should be avoided. Later physicians were not so cautious and hemlock, opium and cannabis have all been tried while physical treatments such as vibration and electroconvulsive therapy have been recommended in the past. During the last century anticholinergics, which are still in use today, were used, initially in naturally occurring forms. Thus bathing in Bulgarian spas where the plant *Belladonna atropina* grew profusely was encouraged, or alternatively, hyoscine and stramonium in the form of tincture or cigarette were used. Synthetic anticholinergics in tablet form superseded these methods and were the mainstay of drug therapy until levodopa was discovered.

Levodopa, which became available for the treatment of Parkinson's disease about 20 years ago, represented a truly dramatic advance and was hailed as a 'wonder drug'. Since its introduction patients do live longer with a better quality of life, but it is not a cure. Although the great majority of sufferers respond when first given levodopa, the improvement is often not maintained in the longer term. Other agents have become available which mimic or enhance the action of levodopa, and new drugs are being developed but none clearly influence the actual disease process. At the present time the medications available often effectively relieve the symptoms of Parkinson's disease rather than cure it or halt its progress.

DOPAMINERGICS AND ANTICHOLINERGICS

Nerve cells whose neurotransmitter is dopamine are called dopaminergic neurones. In Parkinson's disease there is a reduction of over 80% in their number in certain areas of the central nervous system. The substantia nigra in the midbrain, the locus coeruleus and the dorsal vagal nucleus are particularly affected. This reduction in dopaminergic activity causes an imbalance within the CNS so that it appears as if activity in cholinergic neurones (cells which use acetylcholine as their neurotransmitter) increases. It is important to note that there is no actual increase in cholinergic neurones; it merely seems as if there is. Although this is something of an oversimplification of a complex and incompletely understood situation, it is useful to consider the symptoms and signs of Parkinson's disease as the result of reduced dopaminergic activity and relatively increased cholinergic activity. This explains why there are two principal groups of drugs used to treat the disease. Dopaminergic drugs act by enhancing or imitating the action of dopamine, while anticholinergic drugs work by damping down cholinergic activity. Table 2.1 lists the major drugs in each of these categories.

Table 2.1 Principal Drugs used for the treatment of Parkinson's disease

Dopaminergic drugs:

Levodopa

Levodopa + peripheral decarboxylase inhibitor (Madopar, Sinemet)

Bromocriptine (Parlodel)

Selegiline (Eldepryl, Deprenyl)

Amantadine (Symmetrel)

Anticholinergic drugs. Examples are:

Benzhexol (Artane)

Benztropine (Cogentin)

Orphenadrine (Disipal)

Dopaminergic Drugs

Levodopa, 'Sinemet' and 'Madopar'

Dopamine itself cannot cross the blood–brain barrier. Thus dopamine in the blood is unable to penetrate into the CNS and so

9

cannot be used to treat Parkinson's disease. Levodopa gets easily from the circulation into the brain where it is rapidly converted into dopamine, so helping restore the flagging dopaminergic activity. Unfortunately when levodopa is given on its own only a tiny fraction gets as far as the cerebral circulation; most is broken down in the rest of the body by enzymes called decarboxylases. This means that in order to get a therapeutic effect large doses of levodopa have to be taken so that enough gets to where it is needed. Taken in large amounts, levodopa usually causes gastro-intestinal upsets such as loss of appetite, nausea and vomiting. For this reason agents which block the effects of the extracerebral or peripheral decarboxylases have been developed. These peripheral decarboxylase inhibitors (PDIs) are combined with levodopa in a single tablet or capsule; these complexes will be described as levodopa–PDI. There are two such preparations in current use: 'Sinemet' in which the PDI is carbidopa, and 'Madopar' in which it is benserazide. These two levodopa–PDI drugs have largely replaced levodopa alone as the treatment of choice in Parkinson's disease.

Side-effects: Most people tolerate levodopa quite well when it is introduced carefully in a low dose and gradually increased thereafter but side-effects are not uncommon and warrant discussion. Gastro-intestinal symptoms such as anorexia, nausea and vomiting are, as stated above, very frequent with levodopa alone but can still occur with levodopa–PDI preparations. Patients are often advised initially to take their medication at mealtimes. Occasionally an antiemetic drug such as domperidone or metoclopramide is added to prevent these problems. Cardiovascular disturbances such as postural hypotension, with resultant light-headedness on standing, which is fairly common, and cardiac arrhythmias which occur occasionally. Caution must be observed in patients with concomitant cardiac disorders, although in most cases this does not prevent the use of levodopa drugs.

All the drugs used in Parkinson's disease are prone to psychiatric side-effects. Levodopa can lead to agitation, anxiety, depression, paranoid ideas, delusions and hallucinations. Such disturbances usually respond to reduction in dose or withdrawal of the treatment.

Dyskinesias or abnormal involuntary movements are common with levodopa and levodopa–PDI drugs; the more frequent varieties are listed in Table 2.2. They are usually dose-related but there is a wide individual variation in the amount of the offending drug responsible. Dyskinesias can occur in the untreated case but are much more commonly drug-induced phenomena. The most common varieties are orolingual or orofacial dyskinesias. These mouth, tongue and facial grimaces are often the source of embarrassment and distress both to the patient and carer, although others are remarkably unruffled by them. Other abnormal movements include dystonias which may be painful, choreoathetoid or writhing movements of the limbs, myoclonic jerks and akathisia. Akathisia is a generalized motor restlessness which is characterized by a fidgety inability to sit still. After a variable period of months or years of levodopa treatment a significant proportion of people begin to suffer from reduction or fluctuation in response. These problems are described together as 'late failure', and are discussed in more detail below.

Table 2.2 Drug-induced dyskinesias in Parkinson's disease

Orolingual/orofacial dyskinesias:

   abnormal twitching or grimacing movements involving mouth, tongue and/or face

Dystonias:

   slow, writhing, squirming, twisting and turning movements usually of neck or trunk. These tend to be commoner in younger patients and can be painful

Chorea:

   abrupt, brief, jerky, unsustained, explosive movements particularly of the upper limbs which are irregular and asymmetrical

Athetosis:

   slower, more sustained and of larger amplitude than chorea

Choreoathetosis:

   a combination of chorea and athetosis

Akathisia:

   inability to sit still: the individual appears restless and agitated, may pace up and down, repeatedly stand and sit, tap feet, cross and uncross legs while sitting, wring hands or fidget fingers

Bromocriptine

Bromocriptine is a synthetic drug which acts like dopamine on dopamine receptors. It is therefore described as a dopamine agonist. Other dopamine agonists such as lisuride and pergolide are not in common use and so will not be discussed further. Bromocriptine may be used alone as initial treatment as a replacement for a levodopa–PDI preparation if there are side-effects from the latter, or it can be used simultaneously with the levodopa-containing drug.

Side-effects: The main adverse effects of bromocriptine are very similar to those of levodopa. Gastro-intestinal upset, postural hypotension, arrhythmias and various psychiatric disturbances can all occur. Dyskinesias are probably less frequent than with levodopa. Other uncommon problems include a painless digital vasospasm and erythromelalgia (red, tender, painful swelling of the feet and sometimes the hands).

Selegiline

In the CNS, dopamine is metabolized by the enzyme monoamine oxidase. There are two variants of this enzyme, types A and B. Selegiline (or Deprenyl) is a monoamine oxidase B inhibitor, and by blocking the action of the enzyme it prolongs the effects of levodopa. It is usually used in combination with a levodopa–PDI drug and allows a lower dose of the latter to be used. In this way it is hoped that the occurrence of dyskinesias and late failure will be reduced.

At the present time there is a hypothesis that Parkinson's disease may be the result of an environmental toxin. Selegiline given before MPTP has a protective effect in experimental animals, and recent reports suggest that it delays the need for levodopa in man also (Shoulson *et al.*, 1989).

Side-effects: Just as selegiline potentiates the benefits of levodopa it can also aggravate or precipitate its adverse effects. To avoid this it is usual to decrease the dose of levodopa or levodopa–PDI drug when introducing selegiline.

Amantadine

Amantadine was developed as an antiviral agent but was found by chance to have anti-parkinsonian properties. Some authorities would not include amantadine in the category of dopaminergic drugs because its mode of action is not clear. However, it is thought to act by releasing dopamine from granular stores in striatal neurones and acts like a dopaminergic agent. Its effect is unfortunately usually rather short-lived although in some patients it can be an effective treatment for several months or even years. Many physicians use it as an intermediate drug before using levodopa or as an alternative to levodopa-containing preparations in those intolerant of them.

Side-effects: Overall amantadine is less likely to cause side-effects than other agents but can produce various mental disturbances including agitation, restlessness and a toxic psychosis. It rarely results in dyskinesias. However, sometimes it does cause a marbled fishnet-like appearance of the skin called livedo reticularis. This usually resolves on withdrawal of amantadine. Ankle oedema can occur alone or in association with livedo reticularis.

Anticholinergic drugs

Despite the fact that they have been used for over a century for the treatment of Parkinson's disease, anticholinergics have only a limited place in modern therapy. There are several different anticholinergic preparations available but little to choose between them. Commonly used examples are benzhexol, benztropine and orphenadrine. By reducing the relative overactivity of cholinergic neurones they have some beneficial effect particularly on the tremor and rigidity of Parkinson's disease. Many neurologists agree with the use of anticholinergics in younger patients with significant tremor and rigidity, but like their geriatrician colleagues, are not keen to institute this treatment in the elderly for fear of aggravating or precipitating dementia. Dementia in Parkinson's disease, as in Alzheimer's disease, is characterized biochemically by loss of cholinergic neurones, and clearly anticholinergics might make this worse. There is, of course, the possibility that anticholinergics might also predispose younger patients to later dementia, so in general they should be used with caution even in younger patients.

Side-effects: Anticholinergics act on the parasympathetic nervous system as well as on central cholinergic neurones and so impair focusing of the eyes, bladder and bowel activity, and salivation. The visual disturbance may be of minor or no real import to some patients, but is dangerous in those with incipient glaucoma. Urinary retention is particularly troublesome in elderly men with prostatism. Most patients with Parkinson's disease are prone to constipation and anticholinergics are liable to make this worse. A dryness of the mouth is occasionally a benefit to individuals who tend to drool saliva but in others is a troublesome disorder having the secondary side-effects of interfering with dental defence mechanisms and encouraging tooth decay. These four side-effects tend to be dose-related so that if they occur a reduction in dose will alleviate them. The most worrisome side-effects of anticholinergics are the effects on mental processes. They can lead to drowsiness, slow cerebration, restlessness, paranoid ideas, delusions and hallucinations.

GENERAL PRINCIPLES OF DRUG TREATMENT

Starting treatment

The onset, symptoms and progress of Parkinson's disease vary considerably between different individual patients. Therefore there is no single set of rules for drug treatment which will apply to all cases, and there are considerable differences of opinion between physicians as to the best approach even in an individual case. One of the main controversies is when to start treatment. Some authorities recommend the institution of treatment at the time of diagnosis, suggesting that it is more difficult to control adequately established disease. As nobody considers the currently available treatments to be curative, even the proponents of 'early' treatment do not claim that drugs alter the course or eventual outcome of the disorder. Others believe that medication should only be given when the patient needs it because all the drugs have significant side-effects.

Determining when individuals need treatment is based on whether they are handicapped by their symptoms. For example a mild degree of manual hypokinesis may have little functional effect on a labourer but may represent a considerable handicap to a musician or clerical worker. Reduced walking speed might interfere with the work of a traffic warden but be of limited consequence to a sedentary worker. Age should also be considered, although again one must avoid sweeping generalizations. A 40 year-old with family responsibilities may need to function optimally in a competitive field of employment, and so early treatment may be advocated, but if this is done he may be worse off soon thereafter because of side-effects. Conversely it is often misguided to avoid treating the elderly, as early treatment may for instance allow a 70 year-old woman to maintain her major interest in needlework. When to institute treatment therefore is dependent on the needs of the individual, and ideally should take account of the patient's own wishes after discussion of the pros and cons of treatment.

When tremor and rigidity are the prominent features in a middle-aged patient many would consider the use of anticholinergics but observing the cautionary advice given above. In the elderly one would be reluctant to follow this route.

In individuals with early and relatively mild symptoms amantadine may be used as a temporary or intermediate treatment before starting other dopaminergics, on the ground that it is less likely to cause side-effects.

However, at some stage the decision is likely to be reached to institute dopaminergic treatment. The alternative regimes possible are levodopa–PDI drug alone or in combination with selegiline, bromocriptine alone, or bromocriptine plus a levodopa–PDI drug. The other possible permutation of using all three agents is not recommended. It may be however that selegiline should be introduced as soon as the diagnosis is made, in view of its suggested protective effect (Shoulson *et al.*, 1989; Quinn, 1990).

Levodopa–PDI alone

This is probably the most common initial regime. It is wise to start with a small dose and gradually build this up, tailoring the eventual dose according to therapeutic response and occurrence of side-effects. Sinemet and Madopar come in various strengths or formulations. Thus there are: Sinemet-LS; Sinemet Plus; Sinemet 110; Sinemet 125; Madopar 62.5; Madopar 125; Madopar 250 and Madopar CR.

It is usual to start with one Madopar 62.5 capsule or half-tablet of Sinemet Plus or Sinemet 110. In each of these the dose of levodopa is 50 mg. Within a few days a thrice daily regime can be given. It is important that the patient is informed of the strength of medication he is taking as both overdose and undertreatment can be hazardous. It is very useful if the patient or carer keeps a card listing the dosage and frequency of his medication.

Levodopa–PDI and selegiline

As explained above, selegiline reduces the breakdown of dopamine and so potentiates the effects of levodopa, allowing a smaller dose of the latter to be used. It is hoped that using such a regime will reduce the problems that arise with levodopa–PDI agents used alone.

Bromocriptine alone

Dyskinesias appear less frequent with bromocriptine than with levodopa, and some research suggests that later fluctuations in control of the disease are less common when bromocriptine is used. On the other hand bromocriptine does not appear quite as efficacious as levodopa.

Bromocriptine and levodopa–PDI

As these two drugs are at least partly complementary in action the rationale behind this regime is that it allows a smaller dose of each to be used and so reduces the likelihood of adverse reactions.

In the UK the Parkinson's Disease Research Group is carrying out multicentre trials to compare the first three regimes described above; further trials are in progress in many other countries. Hopefully a clear superiority of one regime over the others will emerge but at present each has its proponents and critics. Where anticholinergics are already in use, the dopaminergic regime is usually added, so that the anticholinergic is maintained along with other drug(s).

PROBLEMS IN THE LONGER TERM

After a variable length of time on dopaminergic therapy the majority of patients run into difficulties either with loss of therapeutic benefit or fluctuation in response. These can be described under the broad term of 'late failure'. There are ever-expanding classifications of these phenomena but discussion will be restricted to the more common variants.

End of dose akinesia or 'wearing off'

This describes the situation when the duration of effect of each dose of levodopa gets progressively shorter. Thus for example whereas a patient may have been mobile for four hours after a dose, as 'wearing off' develops he may get only three or less hours benefit.

'On-off phenomenon'

The 'on–off' phenomenon (p. 5) is the term used to describe the fluctuation from 'on' when the patient is mobile, often with some dyskinesia, to 'off' which is characterized by marked hypokinesis and rigidity. The change from one state to the other can be quite abrupt. In some cases the sufferer oscillates into and out of control, i.e. 'on' and 'off', frequently, a pattern of fluctuation described as yo-yoing.

Management

Just as there is no agreed management for early treatment there is none for dealing with late failure. With end of dose akinesia the strategy of dividing up and spreading out the dosages of drugs throughout the day is sometimes successful. This is rarely an effective way of dealing with the on-off phenomenon but is usually tried.

In either of these circumstances most clinicians will try a change of drug regime. Thus if a patient has only been on a levodopa–PDI drug either selegiline or bromocriptine may be added, with commensurate reduction in the former. A change

17

from Madopar to Sinemet or vice versa, or the replacement of bromocriptine with one of these might also be tried, depending upon the regime the patient is taking at the time.

There was a fashion to give patients what was called 'drug holidays'. As the name implies, the dopaminergic drugs were stopped for a variable period, after which they were reintroduced. Considerable benefits were reported, with the restoration of more even control throughout the day, and undoubtedly on occasions it worked. However, in a number of cases the sudden cessation of dopaminergics has put the patient into an irreversible and life-threatening decline. Drug holidays have thus gone out of favour.

The amelioration of late failure is the major challenge in the drug management of Parkinson's disease, and in addition to drug manipulations is the main spur to trials of neural implantations, as discussed below.

DRUG DOSAGES

There is great individual variation in the dose of medication required by different patients, or the same patient at different stages of the disease. Older people, for instance, will often need or tolerate lower doses than younger patients; usually as the condition progresses an individual's dose will have to be increased. Thus one person may be well controlled on a relatively small amount of medication for many months, e.g. Madopar 62.5 three times daily ($= 150$ mg levodopa) while another may require five Madopar 250 capsules ($= 1000$ mg levodopa) each day. For this reason it is important that the patient or carer is aware of the strength of their own drugs. One Madopar 250 capsule is equivalent to four Madopar 62.5 capsules and one Sinemet 275 is equal to two and a half Sinemet Plus or five Sinemet LS tablets. Giving the wrong preparation strength can result in a considerable overdosage or undertreatment with potentially serious consequences.

OTHER DRUGS USED IN PARKINSON'S DISEASE

In addition to the problems of hypokinesis, rigidity, tremor and impairment of postural reflexes which are cardinal features of the disease, patients with Parkinson's disease are prone to a number of secondary disorders. Anxiety and depression both occur more commonly than in the general population, and anxiolytics or antidepressants may afford considerable relief. The immobility and muscular rigidity makes them prone to musculoskeletal aches and pains, and osteoarthosis is not uncommon.

Simple analgesics such as paracetamol or non-steroidal anti-inflammatory agents such as ibuprofen or diclofenac may be useful.

Constipation is a troublesome and frequent accompaniment of the disorder, and if dietary measures with high fibre foodstuffs are not effective, it is worth considering the use of bulk-forming lubricant purgatives.

DRUG TREATMENT IN THE ELDERLY

Parkinson's disease is increasingly common with advancing age (p. 2); although in many cases diagnosis and management may be relatively straightforward and successful, difficulties can arise. Because elderly people often suffer from one or more other diseases in addition to their Parkinsonism, the diagnosis of the latter may be difficult, and indeed lack of response to dopaminergic drugs in reasonable dosage should prompt the doctor to review his diagnosis. The presence of cardiovascular disease, prostatism or dementia may limit the number or types of medication which can be used. Cognitive impairment in the elderly individual who lives alone may make regular drug compliance impossible; those with visual impairment may find it difficult to recognize which tablet is for which purpose. These and similar problems are all too familiar to those experienced in geriatrics; finding imaginative or practical solutions to such difficulties can be an exciting challenge. The use of Dosette boxes for medications, the provision of drug identification cards and large-print written instructions of drug regimes are among the many ways round some of these problems.

SURGICAL TREATMENT

Surgical attempts to relieve the symptoms of Parkinson's disease were first made in the 1930s. Lesions were made in various parts of the cerebral cortex or fibre pathways in the hope that tremor and rigidity could be reduced without causing weakness. Not surprisingly these procedures were hazardous and on the whole unsuccessful. In the late 1940s and early 1950s neurosurgeons began to develop the use in man of stereotactic surgery, which had been used for experimental procedures in animals for some time before that. Basically stereotaxy involved putting a long needle through a small burrhole deep into the brain using careful calculations based on X-ray landmarks, then freezing the target area with liquid nitrogen (cryosurgery) or causing a lesion with a radiofrequency current. Again various sites for the lesion were tried; the most common were in the pallidum (pallidectomy) or the ventrolateral nucleus of the thalamus (thalamotomy). In the years before the advent of levodopa many of these operations were done. They were most successful with tremor but cases of bilateral tremor required two operations, one for each side. The risks of the procedure included a stroke from the stereotactic needle injuring a cerebral blood vessel or a monoplegia when the targetting was inaccurate and nerve pathways were struck. The mortality rate was less than 1% and the risk of serious morbidity of the order of 3% when the operation was done on one side only. Benefits were claimed in about 75% of cases. Bilateral operations were more risky; apart from those mentioned for the single procedure there were significant problems with swallowing and speech, and a number of patients suffered cognitive impairment. Gradually neurosurgeons became more selective, favouring the procedure for younger patients with unilateral tremor unresponsive to medical treatment. This is still the practice nowadays, although the number of patients so treated has reduced to a trickle since dopaminergics have been used.

In recent years there has been a resurgence of interest in neurosurgical approaches to the disease in the form of neural implants or what the popular press erroneously describes as 'brain transplants'. There are two approaches: implantation of adrenal tissue and the use of foetal nervous system material.

Following animal experiments, the first adrenal transplants were reported from Sweden in 1985, the results being disappointing. Two years later Mexican workers described dramatic benefits from the procedure. Since then many centres in various countries have been evaluating the procedure. Adrenal medullary tissue is taken from the patient by an abdominal operation, and a small amount is inserted by a stereotactic technique into one of the lateral ventricles or by open craniotomy. The adrenal medullary tissue is put into a cavity made in the caudate nucleus. Because the adrenal tissue is from the patient himself, this technique is called autologous adrenal transplantation. At present the early reports suggest modest benefits, prolongation of the 'on' periods and reduction in the severity of the 'off' periods in those suffering from the on-off phenomenon. The procedure is not however without considerable risk. Apart from the risks of stroke and cognitive impairment from the neurosurgery itself, the abdominal operation can be followed by ileus. Parkinsonian patients are poor operative risks, and post-operative chest infections can be a serious hazard. It is not clear exactly how the treatment works, as it appears that the grafts do not survive for long and do not produce dopamine.

The other surgical procedure involves taking foetal substantia nigra from therapeutic abortions and transplanting this into the patient's basal ganglia. There are obviously very important ethical issues involved with this, but some experiments are being done. Early reports are encouraging, but there is not yet enough scientifically published material for a firm opinion to be stated.

DRUG TREATMENT AND THE THERAPIST

It is important that remedial therapists are aware of the influence of medication on their patient's performance. Both the beneficial and adverse effects of drug therapy in the short or longer term should be appreciated for the therapist's own intervention to be accurately evaluated and optimally effective.

The undertreated individual may have considerable unrealized potential in terms of, for instance, speech, mobility or manual dexterity which might be tapped if the therapist conveys her findings to the doctor. Similarly undiagnosed depression may be markedly hampering progress in the therapeutic setting and abilities may be transformed by appropriate medical treatment.

Drug side-effects have been discussed in some detail above as they too have important implications for the therapist. Acute confusional states can often be traced to a recent change in the patient's drug regime. Hallucinations, delusional states and paranoid ideas may not be evident at the medical consultation but may well be divulged to the speech therapist who should pass the information on to the doctor who can review the prescription. The dry mouth that can accompany anticholinergic use may aggravate dysarthria while orolingual dyskinesias with dopaminergics may alter speech patterns adversely. Akathisia may present as a general fidgetiness or apparent lack of attention to the task in hand in the therapy situation. The fluctuations of late drug failure, most evident in the on–off phenomenon, affect speech as well as mobility and gait. Thus whenever faced with a change in the patient's performance the therapist is wise to consider whether drug effects could be relevant.

Ideally, as emphasized throughout this volume, PD is best treated by a team approach. Each member should be alert to the possible effects of medications and communicate suspicions of lack of efficacy or adverse effects to their colleagues so that appropriate adjustments to the drug regime can be considered.

ASSESSING DRUG AND SURGICAL TREATMENTS

No matter which drug regime is used to treat Parkinson's disease it is important that its effect or lack of effect is monitored. When levodopa came on the scene, a large number of different scoring systems were devised, and individual researchers quite rightly designed tools capable of measuring the specific features of the disease they are interested in. However, it is worthwhile to outline some of the recording devices which have stood the test of time. Full descriptions are not given but the appropriate references are cited.

The Hoehn and Yahr (1967) classification gives simple instructions for grouping patients according to the severity of their disease. There are four grades, I to IV, roughly equivalent to mild, moderate, severe, and very severe disease.

The Webster Clinical Rating Scale is a method of scoring each of the major clinical signs in the condition (Webster, 1968). Most items have a score from 0–3, equivalent to a range from absence of the sign to a severe case. The items are listed in Table 2.3.

There are of the order of 300 published activities of daily living (ADL) indices which are recommended for general use or for specific disorders. In the latter category the North Western University Disability Scale is one of the most popular scales used in Parkinsonism (Canter et al., 1961; Marsden and Schachter, 1981).

Table 2.3 Webster rating scale items

Bradykinesia and handwriting

Rigidity

Posture

Upper extremity swing

Gait

Facies

Tremor

Seborrhoea

Speech

Self-care

THE FUTURE

It is always difficult to predict future drug developments for any condition. Over recent years a number of hopeful contenders to challenge established drugs have come and gone, but the recent findings on selegiline are exciting. It certainly seems likely that alternative formulations of levodopa–PDI will be developed in an attempt to achieve more even therapeutic effect, as evidenced by the recent introduction of Madopar CR. One exciting new weapon in the struggle to find new treatments or improve current drugs is the excellent animal model of MPTP-induced Parkinsonism in primates. This should reduce considerably the time taken to test out new agents and so allow their earlier use in humans.

If the next 10 to 20 years see as many advances in our knowledge of Parkinson's disease as the previous two decades, there are considerable grounds for optimism about alleviating the great suffering caused by this disease.

REFERENCES

Canter, G.J., La Torre, R. de, and Mier, M. (1961) A method for evaluating disability in patients with Parkinson's disease. *Journal of Nervous and Mental Disorders*, **133**. 143–7.

Hoehn, M.M. and Yahr, M.D. (1967) Parkinsonism: onset, progression and mortality. *Neurology*, **17**, 427–42.

Marsden, C.D. and Schachter, M. (1981) Assessment of extrapyramidal disorders. *British Journal of Clinical Pharmacology*, **11**, 129–51.

Quinn, N. (1990) The modern management of Parkinson's disease. *Journal of Neurology, Neurosurgery and Psychiatry*, **53**, 93–5.

Shoulson, I. and Parkinson's Disease Study Group (1989) Effect of Deprenyl on the progression of disability in early Parkinson's disease. *New England Journal of Medicine*, **321**, 1364–71.

Webster, D.D. (1968) Critical analysis of the disability in Parkinson's disease. *Modern Treatment*, **5**, 257–82.

3

Nursing care

Barbara K. Sharp

Since she spends more time with the patient than any other, certainly in hospital and often in the community also, the nurse is a key member of the interdisciplinary team in any rehabilitative process. The term 'interdisciplinary' suggests a sharing of expertise. This is an essential feature of teamwork in caring for the patient with Parkinson's disease and his family. The nurse not only contributes her own professional skills but is required to maintain such an understanding of the contribution of other team members as to ensure continuity of care for the patient.

Nursing staff have the opportunity to observe the patient over the whole 24-hour period, to assess how the individual copes with the problems presented by the disease, to identify specific needs and to monitor his response to treatment. These observations and responses will form not only the basis for planning nursing care, but will also provide information that will give direction to the therapeutic input of others.

The patient with PD may present with a complexity of problems requiring expertise and support from a number of sources, which can make considerable demands on the nurse's skills in communication and her ability to co-ordinate care in the best interests of the patient.

Most nurses will use a systematic approach to planning patient care, which involves assessment, planning, execution, and evaluation.

Nursing assessment is a continuous process consisting of identifying the patient's actual and potential problems, their cause, and the manner in which they affect his daily life. Individual responses and coping mechanisms vary considerably, and need to be taken into account. The active participation of the patient and his family is necessary to ensure that problems are given a priority that reflects their importance to the patient.

The patient's and carer's understanding of the disease must be established at the onset. The less the understanding, the greater the need for information and advice. Conversely, if the patient and carer have successfully established means of coping with some of the features of PD, periods of hospitalization must not disrupt them, because this may not only hamper the patient's physical progress but may serve a blow to his confidence and self-esteem from which it may be hard to recover.

In planning nursing care, goals are set in terms of what the outcome of nursing intervention will be for the patient. If these goals state specifically what it is the patient will be able to do and the conditions of achievement, then the basis for evaluating care is provided. Undertaken in partnership with the patient, goal setting can be motivating for nurse and patient and give an individualized direction to care, providing they are specific, appropriate, realistic and achievable.

This systematic approach is one way of putting nursing 'models' into practice. 'Models' are scientifically based concepts which form the framework to nursing practice. Different models are appropriate to caring for different types of patients. In the rehabilitation setting, examples of suitable models to base the planning of nursing care would be Orem's (1980) model, with its holistic approach and emphasis on self-care, or the model of Roper *et al.* (1983), which focuses on the individual's activities of daily living.

THE ORGANIZATION OF NURSING CARE

Flexibility is essential. This is especially important with regard to the patient's drug regimen. Medication may be required more frequently and outside normal ward 'drug round' times. The manner in which nursing care is organized must always facilitate and never hinder this. Figure 3.1 shows a simple and practical method for recording the time of dyskinesias and 'off' periods in relation to drug doses.

In the hospital setting, allocating responsibility for a small number of patients to a 'team' of nurses over the period of a shift is common practice. However, in many units administration of medicine falls outside this individualized approach. In the

Figure 3.1 Ward chart for recording fluctuations in PD

Drug 1 _____

Drug 2 _____

Date: _____

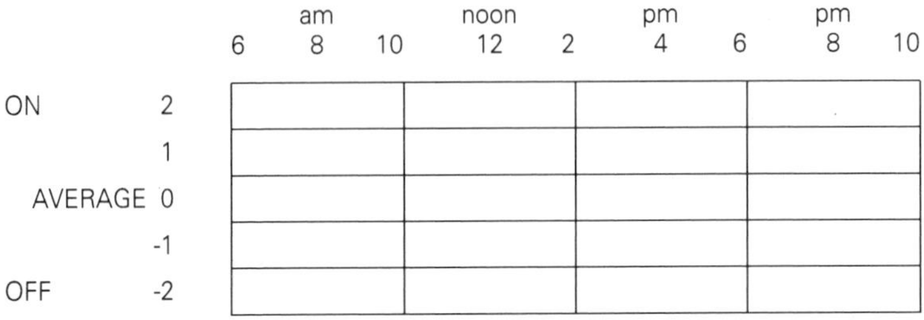

		am 6 8 10	noon 12 2	pm 4 6	pm 8 10
ON	2				
	1				
AVERAGE	0				
	-1				
OFF	-2				

short term, there may be justification for this, e.g. an inadequate number of qualified staff or facilities, but it is always worthy of consideration.

Moves towards primary nursing systems are encouraging. Here, the qualified nurse assumes overall responsibility for the planning and co-ordination of an individual patient's nursing care throughout their period of hospitalization, or for as long as nursing intervention is required in the community. This approach enhances the nurse-patient relationship, and brings the 'partnership in care' ideal closer to reality. Every effort should be made to increase opportunities for the patient to acquire greater control over, and to participate fully in, his own care. This requires a shift in emphasis towards the educative and supportive role of the nurse.

The detailed nursing aspects of caring for the patient with PD will be considered under the headings of each of Roper et al.'s (1983) activities of living.

MAINTAINING A SAFE ENVIRONMENT

Accurate on-going nursing assessment is essential for the recognition of both potentially hazardous situations for the patient and his ability to maintain his own safety. Appropriate intervention pursues all reasonable measures to safeguard the patient without hindering the promotion of independence.

Impaired hand and arm movements may necessitate care with hot foodstuffs and liquids to prevent scalding. Assisting the patient to acquire a good sitting posture, providing appropriate furniture to facilitate this, and utilizing aids to assist with eating and drinking (p. 83) will help to minimize these risks. Initial close supervision can gradually be withdrawn as safety and independence improve.

Accidents occur because of a number of factors, usually a combination of physical and environmental. Detailed advice regarding safety in the home will be given by the occupational therapist (p. 73) and should be reinforced by the nurse. The older patient with PD is particularly at risk due to the sensory changes associated with ageing, so that the incidence of visual and hearing impairments is high in this group.

The instability resulting from loss of postural reflexes (Andrews, 1986) and festinating gait of PD means that falls are not uncommon. This problem may be compounded by the presence of postural hypotension or dyskinesias due to drug treatment (p. 10). Attempting to minimize the risk of the patient falling is important not only to prevent injury, but also because falling, particularly repeatedly, can be devastating to a patient's confidence; so much so, it may present the major barrier to independent mobility.

In hospital, general safety measures may include: adequately orientating the patient to the ward area; ensuring that the nurse call system and the walking-aid (if used) are within reach; giving consideration to the height of the bed, toilet, and chair used by the patient; ensuring that bed brakes are on; maintaining clear pathways for walking; and considering ease of access to the dayroom. The patient's clothing may impede movement or cause him to trip. Particular attention should be paid to the suitability of footwear.

Floor spills in the ward area should be dealt with promptly and dried. When domestic ward cleaning is in progress, hazard warning signs should be prominently displayed.

The patient's lying and standing blood pressure should be monitored and complaints of dizziness noted. If postural hypotension is a problem, the patient should be advised to change position slowly. Elastic stockings may help.

It is very important that any specific techniques taught by

the physiotherapist to promote safety in movement should be reinforced by nursing staff.

The presence of confusion, even in the short term, will necessitate a number of additional considerations in managing patient safety.

COMMUNICATION

Communication problems vary considerably in degree and complexity from one individual with PD to another (Scott *et al.*, 1985). Close liaison with the patient, his family and the speech therapist is required to elicit specific problems, techniques already utilized by the patient in overcoming them and determining how effective communication can be established.

It is unfortunately easy to misunderstand the mask-like facial expression, voice changes and hesitancy of PD as disinterest, boredom or a lack of understanding on the part of the patient (p. 93). These features, their causes and appropriate responses must be known to every member of the nursing team. The nurse must, therefore, be an attentive listener, observing the patient's face and mouth carefully. Background noise should be minimized when communicating with the patient. Periods of short, regular conversation are likely to be more effective than lengthy exchanges, when the patient may tire and feel out of breath (Perry, 1982). The patient should be encouraged to speak for himself and asked to repeat unclear sections of his conversation. The temptation to interrupt and complete sentences for him should be avoided. The patient should feel confident that he will be given time to respond. Some patients find keeping a regular pace of speech particularly difficult. They may have to be asked to speak more slowly as speech then becomes more intelligible. The nurse may also ask the patient to use shorter phrases or echo his phrases to slow him down. It is important to be honest with the patient when you cannot understand what he is saying and acknowledge the frustration that he may be feeling. This is essential in developing a trusting relationship.

Various techniques and exercises will be taught by the speech therapist (p. 94), according to the individual patient's needs. The nurse should familiarize herself with the purpose of these techniques and co-ordinate the patient's day to provide time and opportunity to practise these in a relaxed environment.

We use facial expression extensively in displaying our empathy with others. In the light of evidence that some patients with PD may have difficulty in interpreting the effective meaning of facial expression (Scott *et al.*, 1984), other areas of non-verbal communication such as touch, may be particularly important.

Just as it is important for the nurse to be honest with the patient when she fails to understand him, it is also important that she demonstrates when she has. If repeated endeavours to comprehend what the patient is saying are unsuccessful, it is worth offering some possible interpretations (Perry, 1982) before turning to alternative methods of communication, e.g. writing the message down or utilizing an aid such as a picture board. These methods tend to have their limitations. Many patients experience difficulty with handwriting and cards and boards usually facilitate expression of only the most basic needs. The patient may find resorting to these methods quite demoralizing, but this has to be weighed up against the frustration of not being understood at all. If they are used, the nurse should become familiar with their use.

The nurse must also be alert to the possibility of depression and dementia. These will present their own communication difficulties, which may in turn lead to their recognition.

BREATHING

Rigidity of the chest muscles and limited movement potentially increase the chances of respiratory infection. Prevention lies mainly in assisting the patient to acquire a good posture, maximizing ventilation and encouraging the maintenance of a regular programme of breathing exercises and physical activity, which will be most effective if attempted when the patient is comfortable, relaxed and warm (Andrews, 1986).

EATING AND DRINKING

Swallowing difficulties (p. 98) give rise to the additional risk of aspiration. This indicates the need for particular attention to the upright posture whilst the patient is eating and drinking and to the suitability of food provided. The speech therapist (p. 102) and dietician will provide guidance as to the consistency of food which may be safely offered. Where there are swallowing problems and/or an impaired cough reflex, suction apparatus should be readily available.

PD potentially poses a number of problems related to eating and drinking. The patient's ability to eat, his nutritional state, normal eating behaviour and dietary pattern (including specific likes and dislikes) should be assessed. Independence in eating and drinking should be facilitated and supported wherever possible. Making every effort to ensure that mealtimes are a positive experience can go a long way towards maintaining the self-esteem so essential to the patient's own motivation towards that independence. The nurse should maximize the opportunities for the patient's family and friends to participate at mealtimes and facilitate whatever degree of socialization the patient feels at ease with. The effort of concentration and degree of communication difficulty should be taken into account.

Whilst anorexia can be seen in the context of the eating difficulties described, the nurse should also be alert to its association with depression.

The patient may experience difficulty initiating movements to eat, and there may be an increased need for external stimulation (Norberg *et al.*, 1977). There may also be difficulty in getting food to the mouth related to the patient's postural problems, stiffness of arms and hands and impaired hand-to-mouth coordination. These problems and their management are discussed more fully on p. 100.

The appropriateness of crockery and cutlery needs to be determined in conjunction with the occupational therapist (p. 83).

Assisting the patient to acquire and maintain an upright posture will minimize swallowing problems and the risk of aspiration associated with them. Iced water will help to stimulate the swallowing reflex.

Consideration should be given to the suitability of food provided in terms of its consistency, timing and presentation. In the presence of swallowing difficulties, food of a fairly thick consistency is required. Liaison with the speech therapist and dietician are essential if these problems develop.

Mealtime and medication schedules require co-ordination. Medication is best given with food to avoid nausea, but the patient may require peak benefit from medication in order to cope with the effort of eating a main meal. High protein foods interfere with the absorption of levodopa so it is probably best either to spread protein intake throughout the day or to maintain a regular eating pattern so that drug dosage can be adjusted accordingly (Langan and Cotzias, 1976). Small frequent meals may provide the solution to some of these difficulties. This may also be the best way to provide an adequate nutritional intake for the patient who tires from the considerable effort and concentration required for eating a large meal.

Providing a comfortable, unhurried, relaxed atmosphere devoid of excessive distractions is especially important for the patient with PD, whose degree of tremor and rigidity are likely to be increased by anxiety and cold. As eating is likely to be a slow process, consideration should be given as to how food may be kept warm and appetizing.

Caffeine may facilitate the development of abnormal involuntary movements (Garrett, 1982) by speeding the absorption of levodopa and is probably best avoided in excess. Care is also required with milky drinks which will slow the absorption of medication due to their alkalinity. The patient should be advised that large amounts of alcohol can antagonize the effect of levodopa (although in moderation it is found helpful by some).

Therapy can be associated with dryness of the mouth and a reduced sense of taste and smell which may detract from the pleasure of eating. Oral care should thus be provided prior to and following a meal. This will freshen the mouth and ensure that food does not remain pocketed in the cheeks following a meal.

The patient's weight should be recorded regularly and, when being monitored closely, should be recorded at approximately the same time of day with the patient similarly attired.

Advice and support should be offered to the obese patient regarding weight reduction. Levodopa appears to be absorbed into fat and then released erratically. Weight control will, therefore, assist in achieving the most appropriate drug pattern for the patient, in addition to preventing the mobility and circulatory problems associated with obesity.

ELIMINATION

The nurse should establish the patient's 'normal' pattern and habits of elimination prior to assessing the need for an educative or therapeutic input. Constipation is a common complaint, made worse by anticholinergic drugs. Some patients will be concerned if they do not have a bowel movement every day. It should be explained that a bowel movement two or three times a week is not unreasonable, and that avoiding hard, constipated stools is the important aim. Advice may be required as to how constipation can be prevented. It is important to explain not only the need for regular activity, exercise and adequate amounts of fluid and fibre in the diet, but how this might be achieved in the patient's own circumstances.

The use of faecal softeners or bulking agents may be required by some patients. Establishing a regular toileting schedule may be helpful. The provision of privacy, comfort and ample time for defaecation are important considerations for all.

It should be noted if the patient has any difficulty in managing his clothing for toileting purposes or needs additional support to facilitate sitting or standing. The nurse should liaise with the occupational therapist in advising the patient on clothing and providing appropriate aids, e.g. raised toilet seat, hand rails (p. 80).

During periods of hospitalization, consideration should be given to the ease of access for patients to toileting facilities in terms of location, distance and obstacles to be negotiated.

Whilst incontinence is not a specific feature of PD, it is not uncommon for the symptoms or treatment of the disease to be contributory to the loss of continence, particularly in the older patient. Those receiving anticholinergic drugs should be observed for any difficulty in passing urine. Accurate assessment and appropriate investigative measures are needed to determine the causes of incontinence. It may well be that the situation is not irreversible, but should this be so, the nurse has a major role to play in supporting and educating the patient and his carers in the management of this problem.

Levodopa can cause discolouration of the urine (and other body fluids). The patient and his family should be advised and reassured about this.

PERSONAL CARE AND DRESSING

Deciding on an appropriate level of assistance with personal care begins by establishing the patient's present level of ability in these tasks and the individual's own way of going about them. The patient's potential for self-care should be assessed and barriers to independence identified. It is important to progress at a pace appropriate to the individual. Expecting too much too quickly, or failure to understand fluctuations in the patient's performance, may lead to demoralizing and repeated failure in activities of self-care. Also, anxiety produced by inappropriate and excessive 'encouragement' can make the patient's tremor and rigidity much worse (Andrews, 1986). It is best to work towards a succession of progressive short-term goals. The patient is then aware of steadily achieving a little more and is less likely to feel overwhelmed by what he is expected to accomplish. Each successfully met objective gives motivation for the next.

Adequate time must be alloted to washing and dressing. The area should be warm, comfortable and private. The timing of medication is likely to be crucial to the patient's ability to cope with these activities.

A considerable number of aids are available to assist with independence in dressing. In conjunction with the occupational therapist (p. 77), the nurse should assess the ability of the aids provided to meet the patient's specific needs and advise the patient with regard to using them most effectively.

Facilities to wash and bathe, and the assistance required to do so, should be readily available as the skin is more oily in patients with PD (Holt, 1983).

CONTROLLING BODY TEMPERATURE

Particularly with the older patient, consideration should be given to the suitability of clothing and the ability to heat the home. Advice may need to be given regarding the prevention of hypothermia, due in part to the risks involved with associated immobility.

MOBILIZATION

The cardinal features of PD and the problems associated with long term treatment affect mobility in a number of ways. The nurse must be familiar not only with the characteristic features of PD but open to understanding individuals' presentations and responses. Identifying the patient's specific mobility problems and how they are coped with should be incorporated in the nursing assessment. For instance, if the patient experiences 'freezing' episodes (p. 5), he may already have established a means of regaining mobility; both the patient and family may be able to guide the nursing staff as to how they can best help in these situations. If the patient is unaware of how to manage these episodes then a need has been identified.

It is important that the nurse recognizes the 'on–off' phenomenon (p. 5), not only because it is open to misinterpretation as a lack of co-operation by the patient but because accurate observation and monitoring of these fluctuations may influence drug prescribing (Holt, 1983). Detailed recording of the timing of 'on' and 'off' periods is important (see Figure 3.1).

Encouragement to maintain an upright posture, reminding the patient to maintain a wide-based gait and stopping occasionally to slow down walking speed will further enhance safety (Delgado and Billo, 1988). Turning may pose a particular problem and can be undertaken most safely by encouraging the patient to walk in a wide semi-circle instead of pivoting to achieve this (Andrews, 1986). The necessity to undertake these manoeuvres and the difficulty experienced by some patients in negotiating narrow doorways (Burford, 1988) should influence the choice of ward area for the patient. A number of mobility techniques may be taught by the physiotherapist (p. 58). The nurse must familiarize herself with the specific advice offered to the patient in order that it may be reinforced in her own interactions with him.

Immobility is one of the major risk factors in skin breakdown. To focus attention on the degree of risk for the individual and to take account of all factors involved (e.g. continence, nutritional state), assessment score systems such as the Norton Scale (Norton *et al.*, 1962) or the Waterlow Risk Assessment Card (Waterlow, 1985) will help in planning an appropriate level of intervention. Although some factors influencing the development of pressure sores are outwith the direct control of the nurse, the majority of sores are preventable; this is a primary nursing responsibility. Preventive measures include: avoiding pressure and shearing forces; ensuring an adequate fluid and nutritional intake; maintaining good skin hygiene; and frequent relief of pressure by assisted movement and positional change. Pressure-relieving mattresses, cushions and other bed appliances may be utilized effectively as additional measures.

LIFTING AND HANDLING

There are few situations where the patient cannot participate to some degree when changing position and transferring. Maximizing the patient's active role in any lift or transfer will lessen feelings of helplessness, provide essential exercise and increase the likelihood of an efficient, safe movement being achieved. It can also positively utilize the fact that tremor may be reduced when the patient is involved in purposeful movement. The specific postural and movement difficulties experienced by the patient must be considered in planning any lift. Achieving the patient's co-operation and trust requires careful explanation of the planned movement and details of how the patient can help. It takes time. Consideration should be given to the most appropriate type of lift, the level of assistance required, direction of movement, available space, furnishings involved and the people/equipment needed to effect safe execution. Utilizing kinetic principles, the nurse can assist the patient's movement smoothly and safely, avoiding gripping and grasping holds which create tension in her own muscles and resistance from the patient. Movement is effected from a relaxed, stable base and initiated from the head.

The physiotherapist will utilize a number of different techniques aimed at overcoming specific problems but a few basic principles can be applied in most cases. To assist the patient to rise from a chair, first help him to the edge of the chair. Ensuring his feet are well back under him and apart, his hands are placed on the arms of the chair and whilst leaning forward, he presses down on his feet and hands, enabling him to stand. The chair itself should be firm and appropriate for the patient's height. If the nurse is positioned close to the patient, at his side, and moves with him as he stands she is suitably placed to cope with any tendency to fall forwards or backwards and can guide him gently back into the chair should the attempt to stand be unsuccessful, without risking injury.

Other techniques such as rocking backwards and forwards to gain momentum and leaning forward with hands clasped and arms extended to bring the centre of gravity over the feet (Andrews, 1986) are simple yet effective ways the patient can participate to achieve standing with varying degrees of assistance. It is worth taking note of our own movement as we rise from a chair. This quickly helps us to appreciate the futility (not to say discomfort which may be caused) of 'hauling' a patient from a chair by the armpits!

When assisting the patient to turn in bed, it is rarely necessary or helpful to bodily lift the person. By turning the patient's head towards the direction of movement, positioning the arm across the chest and flexing the proposed upper leg across the other, the patient is prepared to be gently rolled round into position. The use of a handrail or rope ladder may provide some independent movement. Assisted movement in and out of bed can generally be achieved by helping the patient into the required positions as taught for independent transfer but providing the required degree of support at each stage. Movement into the sitting position should be gradual. All recognized techniques of patient handling require to be adapted to the individual's need and the appropriateness of each method preferably discussed with a physiotherapist.

WORK AND PLAY

The patient's working and social life will be affected by PD and progressively so (p. 107–8). Although many adjustments have to be made, the patient should be encouraged to remain as active as possible and maintain as many of his normal daily routines and social contacts as feasible. Different hobbies and pastimes may have to be explored as others become impossible (p. 72). The nursing history should take account of the patient's normal social activity pattern so that advice can be given. The aim should be to support the patient and his family as they attempt to adapt and cope with the inevitable changes imposed by the disease. It is important to talk through the challenges being faced, and to give time to express feelings and frustrations. The patient's family may need considerable support in allowing the maximum degree of independence.

The patient's abilities rather than disabilities should be focused upon, and advice and direction given with regard to appropriate activities. The nurse should help the patient to achieve a day which is balanced between periods of activity and rest, giving consideration to the practicality of this programme on discharge home. Any activities must be perceived as interesting and productive by the patient.

Support groups, involving family and friends, will help increase understanding of the disease by sharing experiences and ideas about coping and encouraging socialization. Patients will be concerned about such things as the time taken to get ready for events, excessive fatigue, experiencing 'freezing' episodes, or being misunderstood by others. Given the right degree of support and appropriate advice, it should be possible to prevent complete social withdrawal.

THE EXPRESSION OF SEXUALITY

PD presents patients with varying degrees of altered body image. Responses to these changes will depend on many factors such as individual attitudes, personal relationships and the reactions of others. Tremor, rigidity and bradykinesia can make even the most simple gestures of affection, such as hugging and kissing, functionally difficult, tiring and lacking in spontaneity (Calne, 1984). Anxiety and depression, however, may be greater barriers to maintaining sexual activity than any of the physical disabilities. Sexual dysfunction is not a problem specifically associated with PD (Calne, 1984). Patients may feel unattractive and have a very negative self-image. They may withdraw from expressions of physical affection due to fear of failure or rejection. The patient's partner may equally feel spurned and find it difficult to come to terms with the seemingly unemotional facial expression and passionless voice of their loved one. Failure to recognize the need for support, advice and, perhaps, professional counselling may lead to unnecessary misery. The nurse can help to promote self-esteem by encouraging the patient's interest in his own appearance and by adopting a friendly, supportive and respectful manner towards him. Every effort should be made to maintain dignity when performing nursing care, particularly when it is of an intimate nature.

The nurse's approach should relay to the patient that she is interested in him as an individual. The patient should be afforded privacy with his partner and family members in the hospital environment. This is not always easily achieved, but some thought to the surroundings and atmosphere could minimize their inhibitory affects on the expression of affection and caring.

Simple gestures of non-verbal communication such as holding the patient's hand when talking to him can help to demonstrate feeling relaxed and comfortable with him, thus making him feel more positive about himself. The nurse can also help by assisting the patient to manage those features of PD that he sees as unattractive or embarrassing, e.g. teaching methods of coping with the drooling of saliva. Some patients may experience a slight increase in sexual desire associated with levodopa therapy and require reassurance about the temporary nature of this. The nurse should be able to refer the patient to appropriate professional help as required and provide information about supportive groups.

SLEEP

Establishing the patient's normal night time routine and sleeping habits as part of the initial nursing assessment will help to minimize the disruption to his sleeping pattern produced by hospitalization. Thoughtful co-ordination of care, i.e. balancing activity and rest and providing adequate daytime stimulus, will help to promote sleep. Patients commonly experience difficulty turning in bed (Andrews, 1986). Techniques for independently getting into bed, turning and getting out of bed will be taught by the physiotherapist. As the physiotherapist cannot be on hand each time these manoeuvres are attempted, the nurse should be familiar with the techniques in order to encourage and support the patient with them until he is proficient and confident about undertaking them. An appropriately placed handrail to the side of the bed or a rope ladder attached to the foot of the bed may further assist independent movement.

The patient may be considerably apprehensive about the degree of immobility experienced during the night; assisted turning and positioning for comfort may be required by some. Simple measures may include providing easy access to a light, to toileting facilities, to the nurse call and items such as a drink, a book, tissues, a snack, etc. (Calne, 1984).

Limb pain and discomfort may be troublesome during the night. Palliative measures such as position changing and massage may give relief but some patients will require analgesia. Bedclothes should be unrestrictive to aid comfort and movement. Providing a quiet environment at night is basic but not always easily achievable in a busy ward and may need considerable thought and planning.

A few minutes of reassuring conversation can be just as important as all the physical measures outlined and should not be underestimated.

Disturbed sleep, difficulty in getting to sleep, nightmares and hallucinations may be associated with drug treatment and must be reported so that medication can be reviewed or other causes considered.

CARE IN THE LATER STAGES OF THE DISEASE

The need to be active in minimizing the effects of long-term immobility has to be consistent and is likely to increase as the disease progresses. As nursing intervention moves towards direct assistance with daily living activities, it is essential to be aware of the patient's remaining capacity for self care and to maintain independence at the highest possible level. In addition to promoting the maximum degree of physical function, this is vital to the preservation of dignity and self-esteem.

In the late stages of the disease, patients may experience an increase in problems such as start hesitation and freezing. The problems associated with prolonged levodopa therapy with their resultant uncertainty and loss of control over movement, can be extremely frightening for the patient. These features may produce considerable anxiety and feelings of helplessness. Painful and incapacitating dystonia may be associated with end-of-dose akinesia and peak-dose dyskinesia (Turnbull, 1986). Attempts to manage these features with alterations in drug regimen may leave the patient feeling that he is forced to compromise between acquiring maximum benefit from the drug and being relieved from distressing side-effects.

Depression is, understandably, commonly experienced by the Parkinson's disease patient in light of the long-term nature of the disease, often associated with progressive physical decline and reduced clinical response to treatment in the later stages. Depression can also be associated with long-term levodopa treatment. These problems are compounded by the communication difficulties experienced, particularly difficulty in expressing emotions. A high degree of communicative skill is demanded in nursing the Parkinson's patient through this difficult phase of the disease. A positive supportive approach which helps the person to relax, develop trust and feel befriended can be crucial to the effectiveness of all other aspects of care. In the presence of multiple barriers to normal communication, the nurse has to demonstrate initiative and flexibility in approach. Techniques such as massage, for instance, could have the combined beneficial effects of reducing stress and limb pain whilst utilizing intact sensory channels.

With approximately one third of patients with Parkinson's disease developing dementia, the nurse requires to be alert to indicative changes in mental state. Practical support with short-term memory loss can be offered by providing the patient with information regarding his medication using large, clear print, symbols and measured dose containers. Medication may, however, have to be reduced or withdrawn to decrease the features of acute confusion (Turnbull, 1986). Appropriate prompts and organization of items of clothing, toiletries, etc, may help to retain independence in personal care for some time. As confusion can be a feature of many forms of illness in older people, the nurse should ensure details of onset and character of the confusion are accurately recorded and that appropriate investigation seeks to establish the cause. Hallucinations or confusion can be associated with the peak dose effect of levodopa in the older patient.

Such is the nature of Parkinson's disease that it will inevitably take its toll on family members. The nurse has an important role in supporting the carers of the Parkinson's sufferer through provision of practical help and advice, by facilitating their involvement in care and decisions about that care. Relatives should be encouraged to express their own feelings and have access to professional counselling.

The various facets of Parkinson's disease can be studied but it is important the nurse appreciates that it is a very individual disease in terms of its impact on the lives of each sufferer and his family. Needs will vary from person-to-person and nursing staff must be prepared to respond accordingly.

DEATH

With drug therapy and vigilance in preventing the major problems associated with immobility, patients can expect a normal or near normal life expectancy. Older patients who remember the days before levodopa may be particularly fearful of the diagnosis (Pentland, 1988). The progressive nature of the disease is such that patients will experience anxiety about the future and have need to discuss this and express their fears and concerns.

PARKINSON'S DISEASE AND UNRELATED HOSPITAL ADMISSION

The patient with PD may be admitted to hospital for reasons unrelated directly to the disease. These patients may be particularly vulnerable to a disrupted drug regimen and daily routine not only because of another health problem but because that problem becomes the focus of the professional's attention. Where drug therapy has to be disrupted to prepare the patient for investigative procedures or anaesthesia, the possiblity of minimizing this should be considered carefully, e.g. are all patients fasted from the same time regardless of where they are placed on the theatre list?

The patient and his carer should be made aware of the likely effects of any essential alteration to his drug pattern so that his anxiety and that of his carers may be reduced when these occur. Re-establishing the medication as soon as possible should be considered a priority. As previously discussed, administering the drugs consistently on time is vital.

It is also important that nurses in general medical and surgical wards are alert to the increased risk of immobility – related problems that the patient's PD will pose, regardless of the presenting condition, and take appropriate preventive action.

NURSING IN THE COMMUNITY

Obviously, much of the nursing care detailed above applies to the community setting. However, the unique position of the community nurse to assess and support the patient in his own environment is worthy of specific note. In familiar surroundings and within his own social network, the impact of the disease on the individual's daily life can truly be appreciated. Response to medication can be monitored and the ability of the drug regimen to meet activity demands upon the patient assessed. Any practical problems in relation to taking the medication in the prescribed manner may be noted and means of overcoming them pursued.

The community nurse has a major educative role in relation to the patient's drug therapy and also with regard to diet, weight control, mobility, skin care and bowel function. Establishing a regular exercise programme can positively influence these aspects of care (Hurwitz, 1986).

The benefits of regular contact with a professional are enhanced if continuity can also be provided. Regular visits by the same nurse are the best grounding for the development of a trusting relationship and enable the nurse to apply her skills with knowledge of the individual situation. The social aspects of the nurse's visit may be especially important to the housebound patient.

The needs of the carer must be a major concern of the nurse in the community. She can realistically assess how patient and carer are coping and identify the need for support services or evaluate the appropriateness of those already provided. Availability of domicillary services will vary from area to area. Where there is inadequate provision, the nurse is likely to find her role correspondingly extended.

CONCLUSION

In preparing for discharge from hospital, the nurse should consider how best to provide continued practical and emotional support not only for the patient but also for his carers. The nurse is likely to be the central figure in co-ordinating and communicating with community services. It may be through nursing staff that patients first hear of the support and advice that can be made available to them through groups such as the Parkinson's Disease Society.

The patient and his family will benefit greatly from competent nursing care. The nurse should also be aware of how much is to be gained by listening to and utilizing the experience of the patient and his carers. After all, as professionals we share their goal of maintaining quality of life for the individual with Parkinson's disease.

REFERENCES

Andrews, K. (1986) Physical management of Parkinson's disease. *Advanced Geriatric Medicine 5* (Eds R.C. Tallis and F.I. Caird). Churchill Livingstone, Edinburgh. 43–51.

Burford, K. (1988) The Physiotherapist's role in Parkinson's disease. *Geriatric Nursing and Home Care*, **8**, 14–16.

Calne, S. (1984) Parkinson's disease – helping the patient with a movement disorder. *Canadian Nurse*, **80**, 35–7.

Delgado, J.M. and Billo, J.M. (1988) Care of the patient with Parkinson's disease – surgical and nursing interventions. *Journal of Neuroscience Nursing*, **20**, 142–50.

Garrett, E. (1982) Parkinsonism – forgotten considerations in medical treatment and nursing care. *Journal of Neurosurgical Nursing*, **14**, 13–18.

Holt, P. (1983) Parkinson's disease. *Nursing* (Oxford), **2**, 448–50.

Hurwitz, A. (1986) Home visiting by nursing students to patients with Parkinson's disease. *Journal of Neuroscience Nursing*, **18**, 344–48.

Largan, R. and Cotzias, G. (1976) Do's and don'ts for the patient on levodopa therapy. *American Journal of Nursing*, **76**, 917–18.

Norbert, A., Athlin, E. and Winblad, B. (1987) A model for the assessment of eating problems in patients with Parkinson's disease. *Journal of Advanced Nursing*, **12**, 473–81.

Norton, D., McLaren, R. and Exton-Smith, A.N. (1962) *An Investigation of Geriatric Nursing Problems in Hospital*. National Corporation for the Care of Old People, London. (Re-issued Churchill Livingstone, Edinburgh, 1975.)

Orem, D.E. (1980) *Nursing – concepts of practice*. (2nd ed.) McGraw-Hill, New York.

Pentland, B. (1988) The management of Parkinson's disease. *Geriatric Nursing and Home Care*, **8**, 12–14.

Perry, A. (1982) *Living with Parkinson's Disease: Part 2, Improving Speech*. Parkinson's Disease Society, London. 26–33.

Roper, N., Logan, W. and Tierney, A. (eds) (1983) *Using a Model for Nursing*. Churchill Livingstone, Edinburgh.

Scott, S., Caird, F.I., and Williams, B.O. (1984) Evidence for an apparent sensory speech disorder in Parkinson's disease. *Journal of Neurology, Neurosurgery and Psychiatry*, **57**, 840–43.

Scott, S., Caird, F.I. and Williams, B:O. (1985) *Communication in Parkinson's Disease*. Croom Helm, Kent, 11.

Turnbull, C. (1986) Treatment of the older patient with Parkinson's disease, in *Advanced Geriatric Medicine 5* (eds F.I. Caird and R.C. Tallis). Churchill Livingstone, 43–51.

Waterlow, J.A. (1985) A risk assessment card. *Nursing Times*, **81**, 49–55.

4

Physiotherapy

Moira A. Banks

Physical therapy has logically been used for centuries to cure or alleviate problems posed by disorders of movement whether of musculoskeletal or neurological origin. Disorders of movement in PD have therefore been the concern of the physiotherapist, and prior to the advent of levodopa, physiotherapy was commonly advocated (Hurwitz, 1964; Brumlik, 1967). The dramatic effect of levodopa in the treatment of PD overshadowed the contribution of physiotherapy, whose use as a therapeutic agent declined. However it is interesting to note that Stern *et al.* as early as 1970 while using levodopa therapeutically acknowledged the value of specific exercise in the prevention or relief of musculoskeletal problems, common sequelae of this disorder. This practice was not universally accepted, and physical therapy in the treatment of PD declined; when prescribed it was generally advocated for physical problems encountered in the later stages of the disease.

More recently there has been a growing interest in the use of physiotherapy for this condition and several attempts to evaluate its effectiveness have been undertaken (Gibberd *et al.*, 1981; Franklyn *et al.*, 1981; Palmer *et al.*, 1986; Banks and Caird, 1989). It is now generally acknowledged that physiotherapy has a role to play in the treatment of this disorder which relates both to the primary neurological state and to secondary musculoskeletal problems.

This chapter proposes methods of assessing the patient's motor problems, discusses possible methods of dealing with them, and considers factors which may influence the long-term management of the condition.

ASSESSMENT

General examination and assessment of the patient's problems is fundamental to their treatment and management. Assessment will reflect the basic pathology of the condition, possible secondary musculoskeletal consequences, the functional and the psychosocial state of the patient. Since the incidence of PD is age-related, it may be necessary to consider also the effects of other age-related pathology.

Several formal systems for the assessment of physical problems caused by PD have been devised (Hoehn and Yahr, 1967; Webster, 1968; Diamond, 1978; Franklyn, 1986). More recently a system of video assessment has been proposed (Kinsman, 1986a), which claims to be more sensitive to minor changes in the patient's state and less subject to inter-observer variation. Many of these systems however aim to produce a rating scale which indicates the overall severity of the patient's state, generally for classification of the disorder rather than assessment for therapeutic purposes. Often too they fail to acknowledge the psychosocial state of both the patient and his carers. Assessment carried out in the more relaxed atmosphere of the patient's own home may reveal functional and psychosocial problems more clearly than when conducted in the artificial setting of a clinic or hospital.

Examination and re-examination should be carried out at the same time of day to accommodate possible fluctuations in the patient's state caused by drug therapy.

Whether any system is used formally or simply as a guideline, the physiotherapist when planning a treatment programme is likely to consider the cardinal motor features of the disorder – tremor, rigidity, bradykinesia, postural instability – together with their functional implications.

Tremor

Initially this may be assessed visually, and since it is increased by emotion or anxiety it may take several observations to provide a realistic record of the degree of resting tremor. Tremor, which as the disorder progresses compromises small precise functional movements, may more objectively be assessed by asking the patient to copy a simple line drawing, to write a sentence, to fasten a series of small buttons, or to undertake some similar task.

Rigidity

This may be tested by assessing the resistance in a limb to passive movement. If a departmental group is evaluating the care of patients with PD in a systematic fashion agreement should be reached on a five-point scale for this response which may vary from severe rigidity to no rigidity. It is known that inter-observer agreement may reliably be reached for assessment of spasticity on a five-point scale (Blake, 1982), and this may also be true of rigidity.

Bradykinesia

This is most easily assessed objectively by means of timed functional activities. Any activity may be chosen, but generally included are rolling to each side in bed, moving from lying to sitting, from standing to sitting, and walking a prescribed distance. Comparable upper limb function should also be included.

It may be assumed that any readings obtained from such activities will be optimal, since the stimulus of testing with the inevitable verbal cueing can act as a trigger which may accelerate a motor response. Nevertheless it is reasonable to suppose that these results will reflect objectively the patient's motor state.

Righting and equilibrium responses

These require a rotatory component of movement, particularly spinal rotation, and the use of anti-gravity postural responses. These normal equilibrium mechanisms are often compromised in moderate or severe PD, and if accompanied by bradykinesia or secondary musculoskeletal changes may result in postural instability.

Such postural and equilibrium responses may be tested intially when the patient is sitting freely with no weight taken through feet and hands. The degree to which normal responses occur

47

when balance is disturbed both laterally and antero-posteriorly may be assessed. Similar testing may be carried out in standing.

Posture

This may be assessed in the normal descriptive way or measured against a postural grid which may enable a more objective record to be made. The overall pattern of the patient's posture should be observed and lack of symmetry or of extension noted. Sitting and lying postures should also be considered, especially in those who are less ambulant. The degree to which the normal cervical and lumbar curves are present both in sitting and standing should be carefully noted since their presence is important in functional movement e.g. the ability to move from sitting to standing. Active and passive range of movement at all joints involved in rotation and extension must be tested to determine the degree to which loss of joint range contributes to the postural deficit. This is the more important in those who have had the disease for some years. Often there is an insidious loss of range of the rotatory component of cervical and thoraco-lumbar movement. Inevitably this leads to loss of range in other components of movement, particularly extension. The converse is true, and loss of extension will encourage loss of rotation. Posture is inevitably compromised.

Gait

Disturbances of gait may often be an early indicator of PD and may initially be recognized by reduced or absent arm swing, general slowness and a tendency to stumble. Often these signs are attributed to 'old age' and their cause only correctly identified restrospectively when a diagnosis has been made. Commonly assessment of gait is made subjectively and this method has had the support of many, including Brunnstrom (1970), who believed that its practicality far outweighed any disadvantages caused by lack of objectivity. Some aspects of gait assessment in PD may however be easily assessed objectively. A timed walk – that is the time taken to walk a prescribed distance and the number of strides taken to accomplish it – will yield both temporal and spatial information. This is useful in considering the functional effects of the basic pathology, since taking a short step in a relatively long time is a recognized consequence of bradykinesia (Murray *et al.*, 1978).

Subjective assessment of gait may include observation of the general posture of the patient, the degree to which arm swing is present, the extent to which he is able to change direction and whether or not freezing occurs. Sensitive questioning of both patient and carer will add to these observations and may identify other features of the patient's normal gait pattern.

These testing procedures may be carried out in a clinic, hospital ward or the patient's home. Increasingly hospital departments have access to more sophisticated testing devices. Polarized goniometry, interrupted light goniometry, or computerized walkway systems may be available. These systems have the advantage of enabling further study to be made of the patient's gait without stressing him by repeated activity. Additionally they permit some of the more subtle alterations in gait to be identified, particularly those seen in the earlier stages of the disorder.

Gait analysis from a computerized walkway system of a patient with early PD is seen in Figures 4.1 and 4.2. Figure 4.1 shows asymmetry of stride length and records temporal data. Figure 4.2 was recorded following a three-week exercise programme. It indicates both increased symmetry of stride length and increased speed of walking. Routine physical examination of the patient had shown slight but unquantifiable reduction in trunk rotation and some indication of loss of spinal extension.

Functional activities

This is understandably the area of greatest concern to both patient and carer. In the assessment of other factors such as tremor, postural instability and gait, many functional activities will have been considered. Others, especially those which relate to the patient's personal interests such as leisure pursuits, may not have been; it is important that in any assessment these are included. Co-operation with the occupational therapist is essential in assessing functional activities.

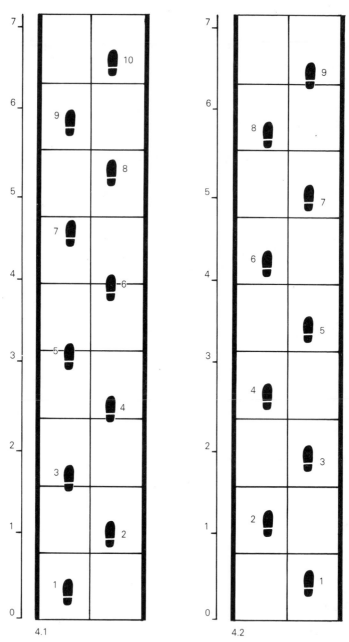

Comparison of Figures 4.1 and 4.2 enables easy assessment to be made of the time taken to walk 8 metres and the degree to which asymmetry occurs

Figure 4.1

Average stride length 141.3 cm (± 6.9 cm)
Average step length 64.9 cm (± 2.4 cm)
Average stride time 1.20 s

Figure 4.2

Average stride length 153.7 cm (± 1.8 cm)
Average step length 75.7 cm (± 1.8 cm)
Average stride time 1.13 s

Psychosocial status

It is generally recognized that psychosocial factors have particular importance in the course and management of chronic physical disorders. Studies such as that of McCarthy and Brown (1989) have considered psychological adjustments in PD, and others e.g. Gothan *et al.*, (1986) have considered depression. The results of these and of other studies have clear relevance for those planning therapeutic programmes. In practice, estimation of the patient's psychological state e.g. the degree to which he may be depressed, his acceptance of an altered physical state, his self-esteem and coping strategies, is generally done subjectively by individual members of the rehabilitation team.

The attitude of the carer towards the patient and his disability is also important in attempting to identify psychosocial aspects of the patient's problems. Such sensitive issues may best be assessed in the patient's home, but wherever this is carried out, both patient and carer should be given the opportunity for individual private discussion with the physiotherapist.

By whatever means it is gathered, information regarding the psychosocial state of the patient and family should, unless confidential, be shared by all members of the rehabilitation team.

Pain and discomfort

Loss of range of joint movement and free muscle action is a common sequel of PD, and is often accompanied by pain and discomfort. This should be assessed in the normal fashion.

AIMS OF PHYSIOTHERAPY

Physiotherapy aims to maintain the patient's mobility, to maximize function and to prevent deformity. When considering specific therapeutic aims for those with PD, it is convenient to discuss them under separate headings, but it must be recognized that aims of treatment are inter-related. Treatment programmes must be determined individually for each patient (Wroe and Greer, 1973), and generally a 'problem-solving approach' should be adopted. The use of a problem-oriented recording system may help identification of factors which are central to the design of therapeutic programmes (Weed, 1969; Scholey, 1985).

The problem list should reflect not only the physiotherapist's assessment but also the patient's perception of his needs. Possible realistic aims of treatment should be discussed and agreed by physiotherapist, patient and carer.

Free active exercise is generally the method of choice in achieving these aims, although other methods may be used. It has the advantage of providing a therapeutic plan which is specific to the patient's problems yet allows the patient to be independent to a large degree of the presence of the physiotherapist. The proposed exercise plan with its implication for the use of the patient's time and energy should be explained and a firm commitment to participation sought.

Most exercise programmes are likely to recognize the importance of some or all of the following: increase or maintenance of range of movement in all joints; awareness and improvement in posture; increase and maintenance of respiratory capacity; general relaxation; and gait re-education.

Increase and maintenance of range of movement in all joints

Free joint movement is important for functional activity. The range of movement at specific joints, e.g. those involved in spinal rotation and hip and knee flexion, has particular importance for those with PD. Exercise programmes must therefore consider these issues. Figures 4.3 and 4.4 show examples of exercises designed to improve trunk rotation. These aim to facilitate activities such as turning in bed and may also lead to increased stride length by encouraging a more reciprocal gait pattern. Figure 4.5 demonstrates one method of encouraging spinal extension. This is designed to improve movement from sitting to standing.

Improved postural and equilibrium responses may also result from an increase in joint range.

Proprioceptive neuromuscular facilitation (PNF) techniques may also be used to increase joint range, promote free movement and to recreate for the patient the experience of relaxed movement unrestricted by the effects of rigidity. This may be achieved by the use of a technique known as rhythmic initiation (Knott and Voss, 1968). In this the therapist using functional patterns of movement passively initiates the patient's action. When smooth

Figures 4.3 and 4.4 Examples of methods of maintaining or improving trunk rotation

On your back, turn your hips and knees, not your shoulders, from side to side.

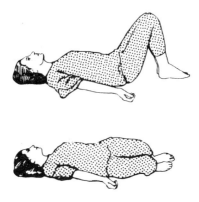

Lying down and rolling over, from the top in sequence, head, arms, hips, leg, first one way then the other.

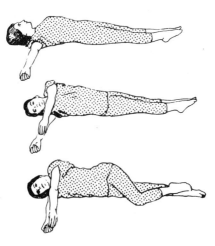

Figure 4.5 This activity encourages postural extension and functional activity, e.g. moving from sitting to standing

Sitting down clasp your hands, bend forward and reach out, then swing your straight arms above your head which stays facing the front.

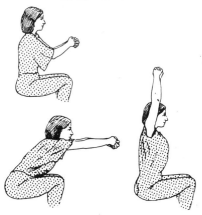

passive movement is achieved, gradual participation by the patient is invited, and gradually the patient effects the entire movement. Classicially in this technique, resistance to the movement by the therapist is applied to achieve a strengthening effect. Some resistance may be possible when treating patients with PD but this should not be used if it results in the patient experiencing a reduction of freedom of movement.

The principles of this technique may be applied not only to PNF limb patterns but to head and trunk movement and others which have functional implications. It is important that any increase in joint range and muscle strength achieved by these methods is incorporated into the patient's personal 'movement profile' and used functionally. If this does not occur it is unlikely that any movement regained will be maintained.

Conductive education has recently become a focus of study and practice in the treatment of PD (Kinsman, 1986b). It is an approach to the re-education of movement using the concept of breaking down tasks into sub-tasks and the use of rhythm and speech in carrying out the task (Nanton, 1986). All these contribute to learning or re-learning an action and carry-over may readily occur from therapeutic sessions to daily activities.

Hydrotherapy may also be used to increase range of movement. The use of rhythmical movement in warm water may also lead to increased relaxation. When facilities for hydrotherapy are not available locally, principles of therapy may be discussed by the physiotherapist and patient and their implementation achieved during recreational sessions in the local swimming pool.

The beneficial effect of hydrotherapy has been noted to extend to functional activities such as speech (p. 97).

Awareness and improvement in posture

Postural problems arising from PD generally occur insidiously; patients are often unaware of change which may be recognized retrospectively. Postural deterioration accompanied by pain, ache and stiffness may initially be attributed to old age, and no attempt made to identify the underlying basic problem.

Assessment will have recognized the contribution of specific musculoskeletal and neurological problems to poor posture. Identification of a problem is fundamental to its alleviation, and therefore treatment programmes designed to consider specific problems will be necessary.

The patient and his carer may need help in recognizing the potentially reversible nature of any postural problem. Feedback – verbally from the therapist and carer, visually from a mirror, and exteroceptively (Figure 4.6) – is important in postural re-education, and exercise progammes must acknowledge this.

Posture is generally seen as a physical state but it may also reflect a psychological one. Patients with PD experience depression to a greater degree than comparable groups – a state posturally associated with flexion. It is important therefore that this is acknowledged and the underlying cause treated.

Since posture reflects both a physical and psychological state, improvement in posture may be associated not only with improvement in movement and balance but also with an increased sense of well-being. Patients often welcome and enjoy an exercise programme specifically designed to improve posture and general fitness. Such programmes may include activities designed to increase postural tone generally and lower limb activity specifically (Figure 4.7) – or to give increased sensory feedback (Figure 4.6.).

Many patients, especially those not in employment, spend a substantial part of their day sitting, and it is important therefore

Figure 4.6 Sensory feedback – important in re-educating posture

Stand with your back to a wall head, heels and shoulder blades
touching it s-t-r-e-t-c-h up tall.

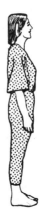

Figure 4.7 This activity is designed to improve foot and ankle function, and therefore gait

Standing behind a chair, legs apart, go up on your toes then
relax and rock back on your heels.

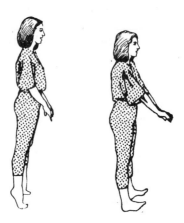

to consider this posture. Sitting posture should be symmetrical, and if the presenting symptoms are more dominant unilaterally, this should be stressed. Care should be taken to ensure that the lumbar curve is maintained perhaps by a small support. The choice of chair commonly used should be considered (p. 74). Low soft cushioned chairs are generally unsuitable for the patient with PD, whose posture is improved by use of a dining-room style of armchair.

If a wheelchair is found to be functionally useful it is important that any chair provided has a firm seat and a supportive backrest. Often both seat and backrest are or become slack and consequently encourage a flexed posture.

Muscles of respiration are also involved in the pathological changes which occur in PD. Movements of the thorax may be further compromised by poor posture both in sitting and standing. Breathing exercises may be included in the exercise programme, particular attention being paid to lower lateral expansion of the thoracic cage. Exercises designed to increase thoracic mobility may well be combined with those aimed at improving spinal mobility, shoulder movement and posture.

Relaxation

It is generally acknowledged that tremor in PD is increased by anxiety, tension, and emotional states. It is also recognized that for a patient the presence of tremor, particularly in a social setting, is itself likely to induce feelings of tension and stress. By using relaxation techniques the patient may be able to influence this vicious circle.

Many methods of teaching relaxation exist and if one does not succeed others must be tried. Methods of 'physiological relaxation' (Mitchell, 1977) which require voluntary contraction of muscle groups to induce an awareness of subsequent relaxation are commonly advocated. This may not always be indicated for those whose pathological state has resulted in altered muscle tone and motor control. Techniques which utilize visualization and imagery may induce a sense of relaxation in a way which may more easily be transmitted to social and work settings.

Those suffering from rigidity and bradykinesia also find relaxation of value. When every action involves effort fatigue is a common occurrence and an ability to relax may often help a patient recover more quickly from resulting tiredness.

Gait re-education

Initial assessment of the patient's motor state will have identified specific problems which have resulted in an altered gait pattern. Alleviation of these problems may have resulted in a more normal walking pattern (Figures 4.1 and 4.2).

A specific exercise programme to correct Parkinsonian gait has been proposed by Handford (1986). This reflects a biomechanical analysis of gait and offers a rational approach to re-education. It is important that an exercise programme designed to improve a patient's gait should reflect not only general biomechanical issues but also individual patient problems.

Abnormal gait patterns may persist despite restoration of range of movement which may have been considered to be the basic underlying problem. These may result from the absence of recent experience of normal free reciprocal gait. With increasing disablement the patient may increasingly lose the feeling of free movement and despite strategies to solve specific motor problems he may find it difficult to retrieve the experience of free gait. Methods of retraining this may be achieved by facilitating reciprocal arm swing and trunk rotation during walking. The physiotherapist may encourage automatic responses at either the shoulder girdle (Figure 4.8) or at the wrist (Figure 4.9). The patient, having experienced the movement will gradually be able to reproduce it automatically.

Another common problem encountered by patients when walking is that of 'freezing' when the posture is fixed in an anticipatory state but no movement is possible. Often patients devise their own strategies to overcome this problem. These may include verbal or visual cueing, or some activity which requires movement of deliberate, cortically initiated nature, such as stepping over a crack in the pavement or an object on the floor. Sometimes temporarily resorting to a different gait pattern such as a high stepping gait will restore movement. The use of rhythm counting and music may also be helpful. It should be noted that these activities enable the patient to return to a more balanced posture with body weight taken on the heel and not supported solely by the forefoot.

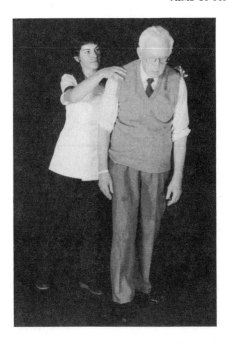

Figure 4.8 Facilitation of gait proximally, at the shoulder girdle

Walking aids

A stick may be prescribed for a patient with a mild disability before technically it is required functionally. It can be of assistance when walking out of doors or in crowded areas, since a walking stick is perceived as a badge which indicates to the public the need for consideration to be given to the user. This in turn leads to increased confidence in the patient, who responds with an improved gait.

Sometimes a stick may be prescribed specifically to assist gait. Unfortunately expectations of improvement are not always realized since the problems which beset the lower limbs may also affect upper limbs and the ability to co-ordinate reciprocal upper limb activity with lower limb function proves impossible. The Delta triangular walking frame by contrast may help stabilize the upper limbs by reason of its need for weight to be taken through both upper limbs. Upper body weight is therefore taken forward and symmetrically distributed. This aid has both brakes and

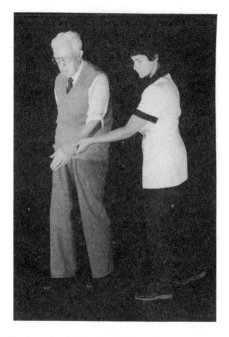

Figure 4.9 Facilitation of gait distally, at the wrist.

wheels on all three weight-bearing points and enables the patient to remain in control of its movement at all times.

Wheelchairs

The use of a wheelchair may be considered. It may conserve the patient's limited energy and enable continued social activity. It is seldom that the traditional self-propelled wheelchair is the one of choice. Generally upper limb involvement precludes its use or that of a powered wheelchair. Attendant-propelled chairs are therefore generally most frequently used. When this is the case it is important that the general principles which apply to suitable seating (see p. 57) are also applied to wheelchairs.

It is also important that carers are given advice on methods of propelling the chair which are both physically economical and may avoid strain.

Self care programme

Traditionally medical intervention has been associated with the concept of cure but in chronic and long-term motor disorders such as PD this is not appropriate; the concept of care is. This emphasizes the contribution of the patient to his own management and recognizes the importance of the carer.

A self care programme will relate to assessment findings and to specific treatment objectives. The patient and his carer must understand the importance of the concept of self care, as well as the rationale for each activity. Agreement must be sought on specific details such as the optimum times of day for exercising, where each exercise may be done, how often, and with what equipment. The patient and carer must be actively involved in such discussions, which ideally should take place within the patient's home environment.

The physical activity involved in work and leisure pursuits should be analysed and postural advice offered. Normal activities which encourage postural extension and spinal rotation may be identified and methods devised which will promote such movements.

Generally work and leisure activities should be continued as long as possible (p. 72). Golf and swimming are excellent hobbies for the person with early PD and should be encouraged. Nevertheless the balance between activity and rest may need to be considered.

It should be made clear to the patient and the carer that the self care programme will continue indefinitely. It should be viewed as an integral part of therapy comparable to medication, and like medication will from time to time be subject to review and adjustment. It may be worth emphasizing that this is part of the therapeutic process to which the patient may actively contribute.

Compliance

In any chronic disorder the question of compliance with an exercise programme and with proposed changes in functional activities must be considered.

Compliance will be more readily achieved if the exercise programme is perceived to be both relevant and realistic by patient and carer. Each exercise must be carefully chosen to deal with a specific problem which needs to be clearly identified. When self motivation is low, the carer can often provide the necessary stimulus.

When considering patient compliance, Lee (1985) noted that specific information is more likely to be recalled and acted upon than general information. Thus encouraging a patient to do a specific exercise a precise number of times is likely to be more successful than exhorting him to 'carry on with your exercises'. He also demonstrated that written information is more likely to be acted upon than oral information. Maximum retention is achieved when information is presented in both a written and graphic manner.

Other members of the health care team are important in maintaining patient motivation and they should also be aware of the rationale for the exercise programme. Close collaboration is therefore essential.

Timing and location of treatment

Often patients are referred for physiotherapy either in the later stages of the disease when clear physical and functional problems are present e.g. pain, loss of joint range or marked difficulty or inability to get out of a chair. Generally by this time problems are established and patients have acquired patterns of movement which are detrimental to their long term management. The optimum time for referral for physiotherapy is when the first manifestation of physical problems is encountered (p. 7).

Subsequent timing and frequency of treatment will depend on several factors, which may include the patient's understanding of the programme, the complexity of the problems presented, and the contribution of carers and others. If a self care programme is the only mode of physiotherapy it may be helpful to see the patient within a few days of the first discussion and identification of the programme. Doubts and difficulties may then be clarified. Thereafter some ten days or so may elapse before the next visit. Progress may then be assessed, the programme adjusted if necessary and the effects of changes in life-style considered. Thereafter further appointments will be at the discretion of patient and therapist, but review at no less than three months (Hurwitz, 1964) would seem to be appropriate.

If the patient presents a sudden change in his motor state e.g. that being secondary to intercurrent illness, a short intensive period of treatment may be advisable before returning to the former pattern. The timing of treatment therefore must be early within the life history of the disorder and thereafter flexible to meet the patient's needs.

Many have looked at the advantages of group treatment, whether from a psychosocial or a resource perspective (Minnigh, 1971; Davis, 1977). Clearly for some patients group therapy provides a stimulus, and they respond with higher levels of physical performance, and social interaction. It is known (Cooke *et al.*, 1978) that those with PD have increased dependence on visual control of movement; without this feedback they show a tendency to drift into overall flexion. Some with PD dislike the use of a mirror to give feedback, particularly those with oro-facial involvement, but may respond to feedback from the postures of others and therefore effect the necessary adjustment.

The success of any group must depend on the selection and willingness of its members to participate. It may be that some become group-dependent and fail to acknowledge their personal role in their own treatment. Other patients may find the presence of others distracting or embarrassing.

In recent years increasing recognition has been given to the value of domiciliary treatment (Partridge and Warren, 1977; Lamont and Langford, 1980) and this service has steadily grown. It has been proposed that treatment directly related to problems in patients' everyday lives is more effective in the environment in which their problems occur (Partridge, 1978); this is likely to be so for those with chronic disorders. Domiciliary treatment also enables greater family involvement and helps to enable specific functional problems to be solved.

In the later stages of the disease the patient may need assistance to achieve movement. Carers may be advised how to assist while still enabling the patient to achieve some independence. Methods of lifting and handling which prevent strain, e.g. back or shoulder strain should be discussed with the carer. Collaboration with others such as the district nurse or home-help, is important in minimizing problems for those involved in the patient's care.

REFERENCES

Banks, M.A. and Caird, F.I. (1989) Physiotherapy benefits the patient with Parkinson's disease. *Clinical Rehabilitation*, **3**, 11–16.

Blake, P.F. Spasticity – can it be measured? *Proceedings of the 9th International Congress of World Confederation of Physical Therapists.* Ligitimerade Sjukgymnastic Riksförbund, Stockholm, pp. 595–600.

Brumlik, J. (1967) Disorders of motion. *American Journal of Physical Medicine*, **46**, 536–43.

Brunstromm, S. (1970) *Movement Therapy in Hemiplegia.* Harper and Row, London.

Cooke, J.D., Brown, J.D. and Brooks, V.B. (1978) Increased dependence on visual information for movement control in patient with Parkinson's disease. *Canadian Journal of Neurological Science*, **5**, 413–16.

Davis, J.C. (1977) Team Management of Parkinson's disease. *American Journal of Occupational Therapy*, **31**, 300–8.

Diamond, S.G., Markham, C.H. and Trecoikal, L.J. (1978) A double blind comparison of levodopa, Madopar and Sinemet in Parkinson's disease. *Annals of Neurology*, **3**, 267–72.

Franklyn, S. (1986) User's guide to the physiotherapy assessment form for Parkinson's disease. *Physiotherapy*, **72**, 359–61.

Franklyn, S., Kohout, L.S., Stern, G.M. and Dunning, M. (1981) Physiotherapy in Parkinson's disease. In *Research Progress in Parkinson's disease* (eds Rose, F.C. and Capildeo, R.). Pitman Medical, Kent, 397–400.

Gibberd, F.B., Page, W.G. R., Spencer, K.M., Kinnear, B. and Hawksworth, J.B. (1981) Controlled trial of physiotherapy and occupational therapy for Parkinson's disease. *British Medical Journal*, **282**, 1196.

Gotham, A.M., Brown, R.G. and Marsden, C.D. (1986) Depression in Parkinson's disease: a quantitative and qualitative analysis. *Journal of Neurology Neurosurgery and Psychiatry*, **49**, 381–89.

Handford, F. (1986) The Flewitt–Handford exercises for Parkinsonian gait. *Physiotherapy*, **72**, 382.

Hoehn, M.M. and Yahr, M.D. (1967) Parkinson's disease: onset, progression, and mortality. *Neurology (Minneapolis)*, **17**, 427–42.

Hurwitz, L.J. (1964) Improving mobility in severely disabled Parkinsonian patients. *Lancet*, **2**, 953–55.

Kinsman, R. (1986a) Video assessment of the Parkinson patient. *Physiotherapy*, **72**, 386–89.

Kinsman, R. (1986b) Conductive education for the patient with Parkinson's disease. *Physiotherapy*, **72**, 385.

Knott, M. and Voss, D.E. (1968) *Proprioceptive Neuromuscular Facilitation.* Balliere, Tindall and Cassell, London, 95.

Lamont, P. and Langford, R. (1980) Community physiotherapy in a rural area. *Physiotherapy*, **66**, 8–10.

Lee, R. (1985) Long-term compliance. *Physiotherapy*, **65**, 1832–39.

MacCarthy, B. and Brown, R. (1989) Psychosocial factors in Parkinson's disease. *British Journal of Clinical Psychology*, **28**, 41–52.

Minnigh, E.C. (1971) The Northwestern University concept of rehabilitation through group physical therapy. *Rehabilitation Therapy*, **32**, 38.

Mitchell, L. (1977) *Simple Relaxation*. John Murray, London.

Murray, P.M., Sepic, S.B., Gardner, G.M. and Downs, W. J. (1978) Walking patterns of men with Parkinsonism. *American Journal of Physical Medicine*, **57**, 278–94.

Nanton, V. (1986) Parkinson's disease. In *Conductive Education: A System for Overcoming Motor Disorder* (eds Cottam, P.J. and Sutton, A.). Croom Helm, Kent.

Palmer, S. S., Mortimer, J.A., Webster, D.D., Bistevins, R. and Dickinson, G.L. (1986) Exercise therapy for Parkinson's disease. *Archives of Physical Medicine & Rehabilitation*, **67**, 741–45.

Partridge, C.J. (1978) Community physiotherapy. *Developmental Medicine and Child Neurology* , **20**, 802–5.

Partridge, C.J. and Warren M.D. (1977) *Physiotherapy in the Community*. Health Services Research Unit, University of Kent, Canterbury.

Scholey, M.E. (1985) Documentation – a means of professional development., *Physiotherapy*, **71**, 276–78.

Stern, P.H., McDowell, F., Miller, J.M. and Robinson, M. (1970) Levodopa and physical therapy in the treatment of patients with Parkinson's disease. *Archives of Physical Medicine*, **51**, 273–77.

Webster, D.D. (1968) Critical analysis of the disability in Parkinson's disease. *Modern Treatment*, **5**, 257–82.

Weed, L.L. (1969) *Medical Records, Medical Education and Patient Care*, Year Book Medical Publishers, Chicago.

Wroe, M. and Greer, M. (1973) Parkinson's disease and physical therapy management. *Physical Therapy*, **53**, 849–55.

5

Occuaptional therapy

Alison Beattie

Notwithstanding the advances in the pharmacological treatment of Parkinson's disease a significant number of patients still experience some degree of disability. These are the patients who may benefit from remedial therapy. Occupational therapy is described as the treatment of conditions 'through specific selected activities in order to help people reach their maximum level of function and independence in all aspects of daily life' (College of Occupational Therapists ref definition). Occupational therapists (OTs) are trained to treat both physical and psychological problems, and apply this holistic approach to the treatment of patients whose problems can affect all aspects of daily life. OTs work closely with nurses, physiotherapists, speech therapists, and social workers, in all of whose fields there are areas of overlap. In spite of the demonstrable benefits of occupational therapy (Beattie and Caird, 1980; Gauthier and Gauthier, 1982), relatively few sufferers are seen by an OT (Oxtoby, 1982).

Patients with PD do not usually experience all the main symptoms of tremor, rigidity, bradykinesia and postural instability to the same degree but each individual presents differently. It has been shown that patients with tremor at rest have fewer problems with activities of daily living than those with loss of postural stability (Gauthier and Gauthier, 1982). In addition patients' ability to perform different tasks can vary throughout the day and from one day to another. While the condition is progressive, the rate of deterioration cannot be anticipated. It is therefore essential that a regular individual assessment is made of each patient, which should cover physical, psychological and social functioning. Relevant personal details, information of employment and details of home circumstances must be taken. The assessment will cover in considerable detail activities of daily living including mobility, personal care (toileting, feeding, dressing), domestic care (shopping, housework, cooking), leisure pursuits and general information about how the patient and the carer are coping with the difficulties imposed by PD. This detailed assessment aims as much to identify areas where no problems exist as those areas where there are difficulties. The therapist should also take into consideration the needs perceived by patients and carers. Equipped with this information, the occupational therapist can plan a programme fashioned to the individual and aimed at assisting the patient to overcome his particular difficulties.

Because of the progressive nature of PD, contact with the occupational therapist should be on a continuing basis, although its frequency cannot be predetermined (Beattie and Caird, 1980). The formation of an understanding and constructive relationship between therapist, patient and carer will help to ensure the most effective treatment for the patient. Changes in the patient's condition and early intervention will assist in overcoming problems as they arise and may reduce the likelihood of accidents. Because of the wide range of difficulties experienced by people suffering from PD, discussion can sometimes give the misleading impression that each sufferer will have to face the entire range of problems. This is seldom, if ever, true, and it is the role of the therapist to reassure and counsel both patient and carer of this and any other anxieties relating to the patient's condition. The psychological benefits of a good relationship between patient and therapist will encourage and reassure the patient and will help to ensure that he performs at the maximum functional level.

The general aims of treatment are:

1. To assess the patient's functional ability and to assist in increasing his level of mobility and co-ordination.
2. To provide advice and support to patients and carers and relatives.
3. To provide, where appropriate, any equipment which may assist in maintaining or increasing independence.
4. To help the patient adjust to his condition and to lead as normal and full a life as possible, at work and in social and domestic fields.

Occupational therapists are employed both in hospitals and in the community. While the overall aims of treatment of both are the same, the type of work undertaken by each will differ in some respects.

IN HOSPITAL

PD sufferers who are admitted to hospital for regulation of their drug treatment or for other reasons may be referred for occupational therapy. The therapist will undertake a general assessment of the patient's functional ability. Sometimes this assessment will be made both before and after any change in medication as an indication of the effect of this adjustment. It may include a timed test for hand function such as the Jebsen test in which patients are timed performing a specified range of activities, e.g. writing, page turning, lifting and placing objects. Testing like this must be done at the same time each day to reduce the problem of variation in performance according to the hour of the day and the effect of medication. Following this, a plan of treatment will be drawn up for each individual. A programme of specific activities with the aim of improving the patient's mobility, dexterity and co-ordination will be planned. The therapist will select social, recreational, and craft activities to fulfil this purpose. Consultation with the physiotherapist and speech therapist is advantageous at this stage, so that joint treatment aims can be established and reinforced by each member of the team.

Liaison between the physio- and occupational therapist will be important in respect of mobility and postural problems. Treatment of these areas which include walking and turning should be given by the physiotherapist and be reinforced by the OT. It is important to identify postural problems at an early stage as it has been shown that these are the major factors in disability at home and work leading in some cases to early retirement (Gauthier and Gauthier, 1982). Recreational activities using music with a clear beat, organized in either individual or group sessions, help to ensure that walking patterns are positive and regular, and also have a psychological benefit.

Problems of communication should be discussed with the speech therapist. The OT should aim to provide opportunities for the patient to participate in social groups where communication with the other members will be encouraged thus reinforcing the techniques taught by the speech therapist.

Writing practice may also be included in the programme. Parkinsonians' writing often becomes small and illegible. The patient should be encouraged to make large letters and to keep checking their size. Tracing over letters or practising recognized writing patterns may help. Where extreme difficulty is being experienced in writing, the use of an electric typewriter or a word processor may prove the best solution.

In order to improve finger dexterity the OT may choose suitable craft and recreational activities; remedial games like solitaire have been designed with pegs of varying sizes. The activity can be graded, becoming progressively more difficult as the patient's dexterity improves.

Selection of the most appropriate craft for the patient will depend on the patient's interests and also on his functional ability. Crafts which require frequent stopping and starting, have a high resistive component, or have to be done fast, should be avoided. The most appropriate crafts are those which are rhythmical and bilateral like stool seating, loom weaving and basketry. Sanding and polishing wood is another suitable activity. Different kits can be purchased which only need to be assembled and finished. The craft which is chosen must be adaptable to the patient's changing functional ability. The advantage of crafts is that they provide an interesting activity and a rewarding result.

Prior to discharge the hospital OT may arrange a home visit for the patient along with the community occupational therapist. This contact ensures joint consultation, planning, and follow-up by a person familiar to the patient.

The organization of sessions for hospital out-patients with PD has had mixed success (Gibberd *et al.*, 1981; Gauthier *et al.*, 1987) While the advantages of such sessions are undeniable, the practicalities may prove a problem. Transport to and from a centre situated within easy reach of all members of the group can be very difficult. Long delays in waiting for ambulances can quickly undo any benefits of the sessions. One very successful experiment which overcame these difficulties was carried out in Canada (Gauthier *et al.*, 1987). There, group sessions were organized and included general mobility (balance, posture, walking, range of movement and facial mobility), finger dexterity activities (including writing exercises and crafts), functional activities (all indoor and outdoor activities presenting difficulties for the group), and educational activities (aimed at presenting a better understanding of PD). At the end of these sessions, patients showed noticeable improvement in independence, general psychological well-being, physical appearance, socialization, and interaction with the family.

Such groups can be beneficially organized by the three therapists combining their individual skills and approaches to the condition.

IN THE COMMUNITY

Occupational therapists who are based in the community, are usually attached to social services, or (in Scotland) to social work departments. These therapists visit patients in their own homes, where a clearer picture of individual circumstances can be obtained. The aim is to advise patients, relatives and carers about the best methods of coping with PD, and to provide any aids or equipment which may help to ensure maximum independence of the patient or assist the carer in handling him. Explaining the problems of the condition to both will ensure a better adjustment and will help in maintaining as normal a life style as possible. Ideally referral to the community occupational therapist should be made in the early stages of the condition (see p. 7). Referral is made by the patient's general practitioner, district nurse or other professional working with the patient, or can be made by the patient or anyone else involved with his welfare. If the patient has been in hospital, contact with the community occupational therapist may be made before the patient is discharged, and a joint home visit may be arranged. As this contact with the therapist is likely to continue, adjustment and advice on individuals' problems will be made as they arise.

Community-based occupational therapists assess the need for major items of equipment like autolifts and also advise about the need for any structural alterations to the house such as ramps and shower cabinets.

ADVICE ON COMMON PROBLEMS

It is the role of the occupational therapist to give advice on the common problems experienced by Parkinsonians which affect the patient's ability to perform activities of daily living and to reinforce advice given by other therapists, for example on freezing and gait by the physiotherapist (p. 58).

The on–off syndrome is a common feature of PD and one which the patient must frequently learn to adjust to. At times he may feel quite well and able to achieve much, while at others he may feel both physically and mentally 'switched off'. The best advice is to be flexible and to learn to alter one's lifestyle to cope with this symptom by doing things when feeling able. This can be difficult, as the 'on' and 'off' spells can be quite unpredictable even on a daily basis.

Fatigue is another common feature. The patient should be advised to do things within the bounds of fatigue but never to become overtired. It is tempting when feeling in good form to take on too much both in the way of work and recreation, but a happy balance must be arrived at, which will vary from person to person.

The question of how much the carer should do for the sufferer and how much to leave him to do for himself always poses a problem. Broadly speaking the more independent the person can be and the longer they can continue to do things for themselves, the better.

Carers can help the patient to maintain independence while at the same time ensuring his safety. For example, dressing, which can be a slow and tiring process, can be made easier by the carer laying out clothes in a warm room. The patient can be safely seated and left to dress at his own pace. However, bathing must be treated with caution, and safety must never be sacrificed to independence. Patients are generally recommended to take a bath or shower when somebody else is in the house, even if assistance to get in and out of the bath is not required.

Independence is a matter for individual patients and their carers. Some people are naturally more independent and some couples maintain a greater degree of independence within their relationship than others. The therapist must try to assess the patient and the carer, their personalities and their circumstances when making recommendations regarding independence. The therapist should then advise both patient and carer as to the areas where independence should be maintained and also the situations where help should be given.

PURSUIT OF INTERESTS AND HOBBIES

The pursuit of hobbies is extremely important for the patient. As well as being valuable in occupying time in a stimulating way such interests encourage social contact and communication with others, so reducing the likelihood of isolation and possible depression. Many hobbies also call for a degree of physical exercise, and can thus be valuable in maintaining general fitness. A study undertaken on the hobbies of PD patients concluded that Parkinsonians are distinguishable by their social isolation and sedentary habits and that people who had enjoyed hobbies and interests earlier in life continued to do so after the onset of the condition (Manson and Caird, 1985). It is therefore important especially in the early stages of PD to continue to pursue existing hobbies for as long as possible. There are helpful pieces of equipment available such as playing card holders and specially designed aids like scissors. Gardening, both indoor and outdoor, is particularly suitable for people with PD as a stimulating activity which can offer encouraging and visible results. Work can be done when the patient feels able, and the amount attempted altered according to how fit he is feeling. Gardening encourages general physical exercise and mobility. It also lends itself to adaptation in many different ways: where bending down poses problems, levels of flower beds can be raised to a suitable height; tasks like planting bulbs, window boxes and tubs can be undertaken while seated at a table; plants which have large seeds e.g. nasturtiums, can be chosen if the patient finds difficulty in handling small seeds; paved paths are easier to walk on than chips. For ease of movement paved paths should be at least three feet wide, or four feet if the patient uses a wheelchair. Some paved surfaces are smoother than others and may prove easier. The addition of a handrail can be helpful.

Among the large range of tools available are some which are particularly helpful for the disabled. The adaptation of standard tools can be done relatively easily. (Figure 5.1)

THE HOME

There is a very wide range of equipment available on the market to assist disabled people in the home. Occupational therapists, both in hospital and in the community, are trained to assess the

Figure 5.1 Adapted dibber and useful trolley for gardening

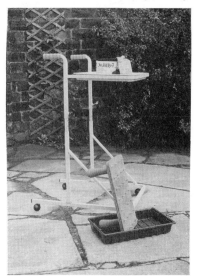

patient and, where appropriate, recommend the provision of equipment and adaptations. Medical equipment shops and even large chain-store chemists sell such equipment. However, expert guidance is strongly advised before purchasing from these commercial outlets. So many different factors must be taken into consideration that it is easy for the inexperienced person to make expensive mistakes.

General

Before dealing with specific locations within the home, there are general principles worth considering. An awareness of potential hazards can go a long way towards preventing difficulties and accidents for PD patients who can move about much more freely in wide open areas than in cluttered, restricted ones. It is therefore important to create this environment whenever possible. Consideration should be given to the layout of the home. Furniture should be rearranged to permit easy access to chairs, tables etc. Hazards like loose rugs, uneven or polished floors, and trailing flexes should be eliminated.

A flexible approach should be maintained to housework. It should only be tackled when the patient feels able and should not be continued to the point of exhaustion. A 'time and motion' study should be made, in order to attempt to reduce unnecessary fatigue. Chores should be spread over the entire week and not concentrated into one day. The amount of effort required can be reduced by, for example, keeping a supply of cleaning materials both upstairs and downstairs. The use of modern labour-saving devices like microwave ovens should be considered. Safety must remain of paramount importance, and the need to bend and stretch to reach articles should be kept to a minimum. Turning quickly can often cause the patient to lose balance and even fall, so it is essential that he becomes conscious of this likelihood and remembers not to turn on the spot, but gradually in a semi-circle.

Public rooms

Rails can be fitted at strategic points in the house where necessary. Grab rails come in varying lengths and shapes. Providing secure fixing is possible they can be fitted in bedrooms, bathrooms, hallways, kitchens or wherever else is appropriate. Although patients rarely have difficulty going up and down stairs, a handrail at the side is advisable. Similarly, rails at the front and back doors and flights of steps in the garden are useful.

The choice of suitable seating is very important. The correct height of chairs can make the difference between dependence and independence. Many easy chairs are low and patients find difficulty getting out of them. A wide range of high-back chairs with arm rests is available (Figure 5.2) which almost always solve the problem. It is most important to ensure that the design, the height and the depth of the seat are correct for the patient. Occasionally a chair with a spring assisted seat may be necessary to help the patient rise.

Problems with balance may make patients feel unsteady when bending down. The use of a 'helping hand' pick-up stick (Figure 5.3) reduces the need for this. There are also long-handled aids available such as a dustpan and a milk bottle carrier.

Where using the telephone is a problem, British Telecom have a leaflet giving details of telephones designed for the disabled. Tremor of PD may make items like telephones slip about when

Figure 5.2 High-backed chair

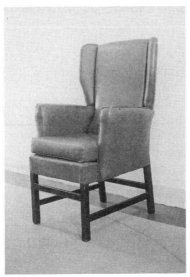

Figure 5.3 Helping hand

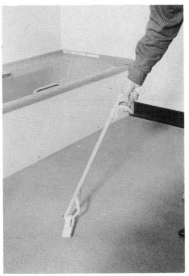

being used; a non-slip Dycem mat placed underneath can eliminate this difficulty.

Bedroom

As has already been discussed the layout of the bedroom must be arranged to allow maximum freedom of movement. Careful consideration should be given to the height of the bed to facilitate getting in and out of it. If necessary the bed can be lowered by sawing off the appropriate amount from the legs or heightened by using specially designed bed blocks (Figure 5.4).

If the bed is conveniently positioned, a grab rail can be fixed to the wall to assist the patient. The weight of bedding often poses a problem for patients. Many find a duvet lighter and more easily managed than blankets. In some cases a bed cage or frame at the foot of the bed can take the weight of the covers off the patient's feet. It may also assist with the common difficulty of rolling over in bed. To date, exercises have proved the best help for this problem (Banks and Caird, 1989), but the aid illustrated (Figure 5.5), which is fitted at one side of the bed has been

Figure 5.4 Bed blocks

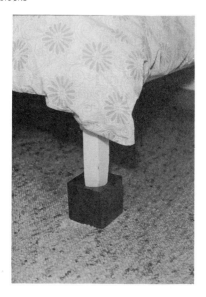

found helpful by some people. Few of the other aids on the market have proved successful, but individuals have found solutions themselves e.g. wearing bed socks and using nylon sheets. A commode for use during the night (usually supplied by the district nursing service) may be advisable to reduce any risk of falling.

Dressing

This routine daily task can prove extremely tiring for people with any form of handicap. A positive and relaxed approach to it should be maintained, and can help to achieve maximum independence. Some patients find dressing is best left until the first dose of medication in the morning has had time to take effect.

The room should be warm and comfortable. For some a high-backed chair is preferable for safety. A small stool may help with putting on socks, stockings and shoes. Clothes should be conveniently laid out to hand and ample time must be allowed for the patient to dress. Whilst maximum independence is desirable there may come a time when the effort necessary to achieve

Figure 5.5 Aid to assist rolling over in bed and getting into and out of bed

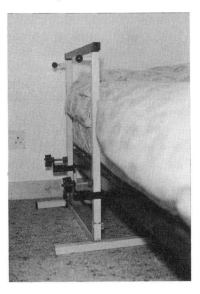

this becomes too great and leads to frustration and exhaustion. Therapist, patient and carer must assess the situation at each stage of the condition and be aware of the need to adapt.

The selection of appropriate clothing is very important. Nowadays there are many smart and fashionable garments which are also easy to put on and remove. Small buttons and other difficult fastenings should be avoided. Elasticated waistbands on skirts and trousers, front-opening dresses with large buttons, cardigans instead of jumpers, clip-on ties and slip-on shoes are all readily available and should be considered. Velcro is a useful substitute for conventional fastenings and can be found on some clothes, mainly raincoats and anoraks. Heavy and tight-fitting clothes are difficult to manage and should be avoided. Loose-fitting clothes in a warm lightweight material should be selected. Leather-soled shoes are less likely to catch on the ground and cause stumbling than rubber-soled ones.

There are few dressing aids of particular use to PD patients with the exception of elasticated shoe laces and a long-handled shoe horn. However, individuals should seek help and advice with their own particular problems.

Bathroom

The major consideration in the bathroom is safety; awareness of potential hazards greatly reduces the likelihood of accidents. Even in the early stages of PD, rails and a non-slip surface on the bath should be used. Many baths are fitted with adequate assistance for stepping in and out. Additional rails can be fitted, the best design sitting across the bath. Many models are available and most are secured in some way to the taps. When selecting this type of rail it is important to ensure that it is compatible with the particular bath taps. When this is not possible a side rail can be screwed to the floor. Some baths have anti-slip bases incorporated in their design, but when this is not the case a non-slip mat, adhesive non-slip strips or shapes must be used. Advice should be sought since mats differ depending on whether they are to be used with cast iron or acrylic baths. A rail can be attached to the wall at the side of the bath but it is important to ensure that it is securely fitted and at the most convenient height for the patient. Its use is limited to steadying the patient when stepping in and out.

Figure 5.6 Bath seat, board, and mat

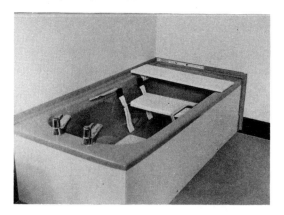

Although for the majority of patients a bath rail and mat are sufficient, some require further help. The use of bath boards in conjunction with bath seats may solve the problem for some people (Figure 5.6). To use these the patient sits on the board, swings his legs over the bath, slides along the board and lowers himself onto the seat and reverses the process when getting out. Again, expert advice should be sought as some bath seats are unsuitable and dangerous when used with acrylic baths.

More expensive power-operated seats are available. One is particularly useful, the Mangar Bath Lift, which raises the patient by means of bellows operated by a compressor unit. Regardless of which bath aids are used, it is always advisable to drain the water before stepping out. Also, as a further precaution, a carer or relative should be in the house when a bath is taken, even if their assistance is not required. Where none of the above aids are adequate, special hoists like the Autolift are available, but their use is frequently restricted by their size.

Alternatively, a shower can be used. This may either be a separate unit or fitted over the bath. With the latter, difficulty may be experienced in stepping over the side of the bath. A grab rail fitted to the wall can give support when standing in the shower or the patient can sit on a specially designed slatted bath board. Alternatively a swivel bather could be used (Figure 5.7).

Figure 5.7 Swivel bather

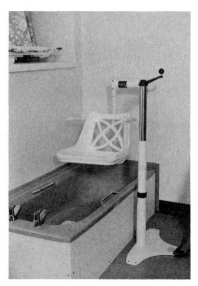

In cases of extreme difficulty a shower cabinet may be the only solution, but this is expensive and may prove impossible to fit in the available space. The patient should use one of the seats available for these cabinets.

Problems with sitting on and rising from the toilet can be overcome by securely fitted rails. The temptation to hold onto fitments like towel rails and toilet roll holders should be avoided as this can lead to accidents. There is a wide range of different rails available. Grab rails can be fitted to the wall at the side of the toilet at the most appropriate height for the patient (Figure 5.8). Numerous other appliances are on the market. Frames which fit round the toilet can either be free-standing or screwed to the floor, the latter being considerably more stable. Other rails can be attached to the wall behind the toilet. Some models are permanently in place and others can be folded up against the wall. If the toilet is too low for the patient a raised seat may be required. These are made in different heights, and it is important to select the correct one.

A seat or perching stool may be useful when the patient is washing in order to reduce fatigue. Shaving can prove a problem

Figure 5.8 Wall-mounted toilet rails, grab rail and folding rail

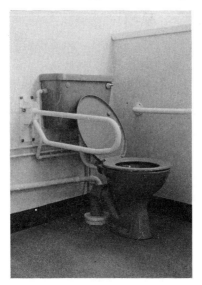

and the use of an electric shaver may help. Re-chargeable models are particularly suitable.

Kitchen

The major factor in the kitchen is again safety, and the layout should reflect this. Open space is required for ease of movement and work surfaces should be planned so that carrying is reduced to a minimum. This is particularly important between cooker and sink in order that pans can be slipped from one to the other. An electric kettle is best situated near the sink with items like tea and coffee beside it. A lightweight jug can be kept to fill the kettle, and a kettle tipper can be used. When cooking potatoes and other vegetables a wire basket (Figure 5.9) placed inside the pot eliminates the need to drain boiling water. The use of a cooker guard is an additional precaution. Simple equipment such as a trolley can greatly reduce journeys to and from the kitchen. A range of trolleys specially designed for the disabled is readily available (Figure 5.10). Some models have

Figure 5.9 Wire cooking basket. Also shown is cooker safety guard rail

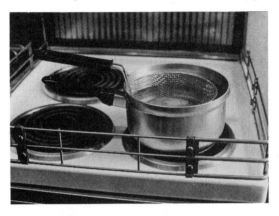

Figure 5.10 Trolley

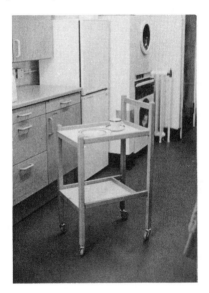

a half-sized lower shelf so that they can be turned side on and used as a table.

General muscular weakness can make certain tasks impossible like undoing jars and bottles and turning taps on and off. Electric gadgets like can-openers can also prove useful, but it is essential to try them first, as some models are better than others. Wall-mounted can-openers are sometimes more suitable than electric ones.

Chores in the kitchen should be carefully planned to reduce unnecessary fatigue and should only be undertaken when the patient feels able. Many modern convenience foods can be used when the patient does not feel up to preparing and cooking. A supply should be kept for such unpredictable occasions. An adjustable perching stool is useful and can be employed when baking, washing dishes, and ironing. Unbreakable bowls and plates are helpful, and the use of a Dycem mat will prevent slipping.

A fully automatic washing machine greatly assists with laundry, and the choice of non-iron materials and fabric softener reduces the need to iron. A tumble dryer also helps minimize ironing.

Shopping

This should be planned to suit the individual. Frequent short visits may be better than major shopping trips. The choice of shops and the facilities they offer should be considered. Thus, a supermarket with well-designed trolleys, open-spaced aisles, and assistance with packing and loading is of great value. Also helpful are shops which undertake home deliveries.

Problems of feeding should be discussed with the speech therapist (p. 98), who will advise on difficulties of swallowing, and also on the most appropriate choice of food as it is essential that the patient has a nutritious and well-balanced diet. If necessary special cutlery and plates can be provided by the occupational therapist.

Feeding

Problems of feeding can result in embarrassment and a feeling of self-consciousness which may lead to isolation (p. 98). It is therefore important to find a solution to this problem.

Tremor and poor grip can give rise to difficulties with eating. The challenge of a plate of soup has proved too much for some patients, who wisely opt to use a mug! Because of problems in swallowing some patients find difficulty in coping with chunky pieces of food and so have to alter their diet. Such adaptations of normal eating habits are sensible and can overcome difficulties, but in addition there are specially designed cutlery, plates and mats.

There are several different sets of cutlery available but the Sunflower range with its large handles and easy-to-grip surfaces has proved useful. Tremor can cause food to scatter and plates to slide. The use of non-slip Dycem mats under plates is extremely effective. These mats come in different shapes and sizes and can be placed on trays and trolleys. Plates with raised lips help to prevent spillage. They come either in crockery (the Doulton range) or unbreakable plastic (the Manoy range). Mugs which are specially designed and easy to grip are also available in both ranges. Half-filled mugs may also reduce the likelihood of spillage. In the event of extreme difficulty with drinking, flexible straws or mugs with lids can be used. Experimentation with the height of table and chair may help to overcome difficulties by reducing the distance from plate to mouth.

REFERRAL TO OCCUPATIONAL THERAPY

In hospital, patients are referred to occupational therapy by the doctors looking after them. However, in the community referral can be made by any medical person, relative, friend or even the patient himself, but waiting lists may be long. Some local branches of the PDS have OTs attached to them and advantage should be taken of their availability and skills.

Further help with choice of special equipment is available from the addresses listed in the Appendix, but expert advice is strongly advised if purchasing. However it should be borne in mind that equipment is not always necessarily a solution, as reorganization and planning is often sufficient.

REFERENCES

Banks, M.A. and Caird, F.I. (1989) Physiotherapy benefits the patient with Parkinson's disease. *Clinical Rehabilitation*, **3**, 11–16.

Beattie, A. and Caird, F.I. (1980) The occupational therapist and the patient with Parkinson's disease. *British Medical Journal*, **280**, 1354–55.

Gauthier, L. and Gauthier, S. (1982) Activities of daily living in Parkinson's disease, in *Proceedings of the 8th International Congress World Federation of Occupational Therapists*, Hamburg, Germany, pp. 589–93.

Gauthier, L., Dalziel, S. and Gauthier, S. (1987) The benefits of group occupational therapy for patients with Parkinson's disease. *American Journal of Occupational Therapy*, **41**, 360–5.

Gauthier, L. and Gauthier S. (1987) Functional rehabilitation of patients with Parkinson's disease. *Physiotherapy Canada*, **35**, 220–22.

Gibberd, F.B., Page, W.G.R., Spencer, K.M., Kinnear, E., Hawksworth, J.B. (1981) Controlled trial of physiotherapy and occupational therapy for Parkinson's disease. *British Medical Journal*, **282**, 1196.

Manson, L., Caird, F.I. (1985) Survey of the hobbies and transport of patients with Parkinson's disease. *British Journal of Occupational Therapy*, **48**, 199.

Oxtoby, M. (1982) *Parkinson's disease Patients and their Social Needs*. Parkinson's Disease Society, London.

FURTHER READING

Beattie, A. (1981) Aids to daily living for the patient with Parkinson's disease. *British Journal of Occupational Therapy*, **44**, 53–5.

Davis, J.C. (1977) Team Management of Parkinson's disease. *American Journal of Occupational Therapy*, **31**, 300–8.

Franklyn, S., Perry, A. and Beattie, A. (1982) *Living with Parkinson's disease*. Parkinson's Disease Society, London.

Helm, M. (1987) *Occupational Therapy with the Elderly*. Churchill Livingstone, Edinburgh, 79–84.

Mutch, W.J., Swallow, M.W., Baker, M., Beasley, J. and Oxtoby, M. (1989) A pilot study of patient rated disability and the need for aids in Parkinson's disease. *Clinical Rehabilitation*, **3**, 151–5.

Oxtoby, M., Findley, L., Kelson, N., *et al.* (1988) A strategy for the management of Parkinson's disease and the long-term support of patients and their carers. End of pilot report. Parkinson's Disease Society, London.

Tromly, C.A. and Scott, A.D (1977) *Occupational therapy for physical dysfunction*, Williams and Wilkins, Baltimore.

Turner, A. (1987) *The Practice of Occupational Therapy*. Churchill Livingstone, Edinburgh.

Weiner, W.J., Singer, C. (1989) Parkinson's disease and nonpharmacologic treatment programs. *Journal of American Geriatric Society*, **37** 359–53.

Hopkins, H.L. and Smith, H.D. (1983) *Willard and Spackman's Occupational Therapy* (6th edn), 405–7.

6

Speech therapy

Sheila Scott

'Parkinson's disease results in a world of decreasing communicative opportunities'.
(Speech Therapy Working Party of Parkinson's Disease
Society, 1988)

For too long speech therapists accepted the limited numbers of referrals of PD sufferers, so perpetuating the opinion of many doctors that speech therapy had little to offer. Speech therapy assessment was generally considered of value pre- and post-operatively, and prior to changes in drug regime. Referral for active therapy was controversial, as the benefits were considered to be limited and treatment thus a waste of valuable speech therapist's time. Research over the last ten years has done much to dispel these myths, and has convinced many speech therapists and others that there is considerable value in the treatment of PD. It has also in a small way encouraged the medical profession to give the speech therapists a proper role in the management of the disease (Scott and Caird, 1981, 1984; Robertson and Thomson, 1984; Scott *et al.*, 1985).

THE CHARACTERISTICS OF PARKINSONIAN SPEECH

'The struggle to communicate is lost before he has even uttered a word'. Robertson (1988) thus encapsulates the sense of isolation and uselessness encountered by the sufferer. The loss of facial expression falsely implies a person who is bored, apathetic, or even worse, of low intelligence. Rigidity inhibits his use of gesture, and the stooped posture, by reducing eye contact, does little to impress the listener. Stooping may also heighten the problem of drooling, and increase the poor self-image. All these difficulties and not a word uttered.

The problems listed in Table 6.1 are traditionally considered those of a hypokinetic dysarthria (Darley, Aronson and Brown,

Table 6.1 Speech characteristics of Parkinson's disease

	Abnormal manifestations
Pitch:	Disordered pitch levels, loss of variation
Volume	Loss of controlled variation quiet, monoloudness, fading
Rate	Short bursts of variable rate inappropriate silences
Intonation	Monotonous speech and lacking expression
Rhythm	Flattened, reduced stress
Articulatory precision	Reduced lip movement, occasional slurring

1975), but Scott *et al.* (1983) regard the term dysprosody as more appropriate, particularly because it focuses therapy. Prosody is defined as that aspect of spoken language that consists of the correct placing of stress, pitch, and tone upon syllables and words. It is obviously dependent upon a well-controlled respiratory and phonational system, and it has been argued that the term dysarthria is therefore correct and appropriate. However 'dysarthria' focuses on the mechanical aspects of speech, and therapeutically leaves the prosodic aspects as 'the icing on the cake'.

Variations in prosody can have dramatic effects on speech. The listener expects certain features for English, and the irregular use of rhythm, distorted voicing and intonation impair intelligibility and gives the impression of incompetent articulation. Prosodic variations can have a significant effect on the meaning of speech, and many fluent speakers use aspects of prosody as a sort of verbal shorthand (Table 6.2). These features are lost to the Parkinsonian. By concentrating attention on them, a method of therapy has been devised which can bring about dramatic improvements in speech in many patients (Scott *et al.*, 1983).

Table 6.2 Prosodic functions

1. 'It's me, Sheila'
   Nominative function, i.e. Me and Sheila in apposition, compared with:

   'It's me, Sheila'
   Vocative function, i.e. Me and Sheila as different people

2. 'Don't hurry'
   Sarcasm, compared with:

   'Don't hurry'
   Caring advice

3. Or an elliptical form
   'Coffee?'
   Using a rising intonation to imply, 'Do you want coffee?'

Speech disorder is common in PD, may occasionally be the major source of difficulty (Critchley, 1981), and is responsible for some of most upsetting and isolating aspects of the disease (Oxtoby, 1982). It is generally accepted that speech disorder occurs in half of all cases, and that it becomes commoner as the disease progresses (Uziel *et al.*, 1975). In two recent surveys (Oxtoby, 1982; Mutch *et al.*, 1986), only 3–4% of sufferers are recorded as having had received speech therapy, though between 43 and 65% felt they needed it.

Respiration

Objective assessments of respiration reveal inflexible and shallow breathing patterns, reduced lung capacity, and poor control and loss of synchrony between respiration and phonation (Darley, Aronson and Brown, 1975). There is a wastage of air before an utterance, and a tailing off, or running out of breath before the end of the phrase. An adequate expiratory air flow is vital to sustain voice and produce speech. The reduction in respiratory function found in as many as 87% of PD patients (Robertson, 1988), is attributed to rigidity of the chest musculature (Kim, 1968; Mueller 1971).

Phonation

Poor respiratory function has a direct influence on phonation. Darley, Aronson and Brown (1975) consider that one of the most salient features of the Parkinsonian speech disorder is in the phonatory aspects of speech. Canter (1963) reported the difficulties PD patients have in achieving both the delicate control over subglottic pressure necessary for quiet phonation, and the same degrees of loudness as age-matched normals. Voice is difficult to initiate and a reduced vocal level is a significant feature, as shown by Johnson (1988), who used the Cirrus sound level meter and the Jedcom vocal loudness indicator both in assessment and as therapeutic tools. After a period of self-monitoring with the Jedcom indicator, there were significant changes in loudest volume, mean volume in reading, and particularly in the range of volume achieved. However, since reduced vocal loudness is a feature of depression, which is common in PD (Gotham *et al.*, 1986), further study is clearly desirable.

Parkinson's disease patients have a reduced variability in pitch, and use a restricted range of pitch levels (Canter, 1965a, b; Kammermeier, 1969). Recent studies by Robertson (1988; Figure 6.1) used the Glottal Frequency Analyser (GFA 60), which measures the fundamental frequency of the voice during speech, and gives objective and reliable measurements of the mean pitch and range of pitch of the voice. Parkinsonians have a narrower pitch range than normals of a similar age, and for 60–80% of the time use a maximum range of one half semitone. This study provides valuable information on the monotonous quality of their voice, and highlights their inability to maximize their potential pitch range. Robertson is now using the GFA as a therapeutic tool, and it is proving valuable in reducing the monotonous quality of the voice.

Articulation

Articulatory accuracy declines with age (Ryan and Burke, 1974), owing to the general effects of ageing on the neuromusculature, or inadequate proprioception (Hutchinson and Beasley, 1976). Although articulation in PD is often described as slurred and imprecise, and has been the subject of much study, assessment of phonemes in isolation reveals no apparent difficulty. However,

Figure 6.1 Glottal Frequency Analyser printouts from patient with PD (L) and normal (R)

GLOTTAL
FREQUENCY ANALYSER

DATE OF TEST: 19 - 1 - 87

NAME: C.T. (M)

NUMBER: P.D. 1

SOURCE: EGG
TRUNCATION: YES

DISTRIBUTION:

MEAN PITCH: 121 HERTZ
RANGE: 3, 7 SEMITONES

GLOTTAL
FREQUENCY ANALYSER

DATE OF TEST: 19 - 1 - 87

NAME: B.T. (F)

NUMBER: NORM

SOURCE: EGG
TRUNCATION: YES

DISTRIBUTION:

MEAN PITCH: 197 HERTZ
RANGE: 4, 6 SEMITONES

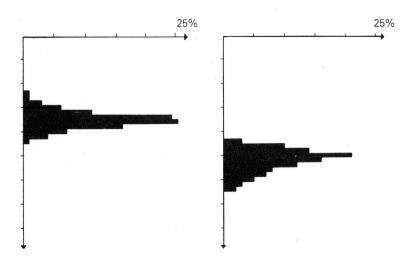

FREQ.	%	FREQ.	%	FREQ.	%		FREQ.	%	FREQ.	%	FREQ.	%
46.		104.	6	233.			46.		104.		233.	7
49.		110.	11	247.			49.		110.		247.	5
52.		117.	24	262.			52.		117.		262.	3
55.		123.	25	277.			55.		123.		277.	2
58.		131.	16	294.			58.		131.		294.	
62.		139.	7	311.			62.		139.		311.	
65.		147.	4	330.			65.		147.		330.	
69.		156.	1	349.			69.		156.	3	349.	
73.		165.		370.			73.		165.	10	370.	
78.		175.		392.			78.		175.	14	392.	
82.		185.		415.			82.		185.	21	415.	
87.	1	196.		440.			87.		196.	16	440.	
93.	1	208.		466.			93.		208.	12	466.	
98.	3	220.		494.			98.		220.	8	494.	

in continuous speech precision deteriorates. This may be attributed to the disordered prosody giving an impression of slurring. Articulatory contacts are reduced, because the lower volume and control of the air stream affects the intensity of plosive and fricative production. This is also well documented as a feature of ageing (Ptacek *et al.*, 1966). The loss of breath control influences rate, and by affecting the control over phoneme production causes elison of phonemes and syllables. Incomplete sound production and continuous voicing, together with clustering of phonemes and lack of pausing may give the impression of interference with rate (Weismer, 1984; Robertson, 1988).

Prosody

Speech hesitations and repetitions are common features of ageing. Scott *et al.* (1985) consider that the use of elliptical speech, sarcasm, and abstract humour decline with age. However the normal elderly do not completely lose the use of these features, or lose the ability to discriminate their use, in the speech of others. The PD sufferer does seem to lose this ability, his ability to imitate certain forms of stressing, and to match the appropriate speech form to facial expressions. It is not surprising that many assume that these inappropriate responses, together with their rapid mumbling speech, are signs of loss of intellect.

Drug therapy

Effective drug therapy stabilizes many patients' symptoms and can benefit speech. In many cases improvement in speech is the first sign of a response to treatment (Judge and Caird, 1977). Most studies of the influence of drugs on speech have been carried out with levodopa preparations (Rigrodsky and Morrison, 1970; Mawdsley and Gamsu, 1971). Levodopa improves intelligibility in most patients, and normalizes the electromyographic pattern of the labial muscles, and the speed and symmetry of labial function (Nakano *et al.*, 1973). Although improvements in speech are not as dramatic as the physical gains produced by treatment, they are significant.

When orofacial dyskinesia develops (p. 11), speech may

become unintelligible owing to akinesia and dysphonia (Marsden and Parkes, 1976). Though sufferers may tolerate the resulting distress because the drug works, it is the cause of much anguish for families and carers, and can be yet another cause of social breakdown.

There appear to have been no specific studies of the effects on speech of other anti-Parkinsonian drugs, but the general effects of these and other drugs which many influence speech have been reviewed (Gawel, 1981; Scott, Caird, and Williams, 1985).

THE SOCIAL CONSEQUENCES OF THE SPEECH DISORDER

Sufferer, relatives, and carers may incorrectly accept that a decrease in daily activity and a more passive life-style are part of the disease. Sufferers may lose confidence in their social abilities, in part because of their increasingly limited physical and communicative skills. The latter leads to loss of privacy, and because he is dependent on another to communicate his needs for him, he loses control of his environment. This increased dependence often leads to withdrawal and social isolation, as loss of confidence causes an ever-decreasing spiral of frustration and despondency.

Too often the carer's acceptance of the disorder results from lack of knowledge of its nature, and much may also be attributed to the effects of ageing. Attempts to overprotect and mother the sufferer cause loss of status, which does little to alleviate the already fraught situation. It may be many years before activities of daily life are compromised, and the sufferer should be encouraged to keep up an active role in running the home (Parkes, 1982). If there is a need to adjust to the more serious effects of the disease, then there must be an enormous effort to keep social activities alive. People not given the opportunity to talk, lose the will to communicate which it is vital to keep alive (Butfield, 1961).

Physical and communicative handicaps may have an alarming effect on the sufferer's vocal image. Listeners treat him differently, believing that his personality must have changed. They misunderstand the 'on and off' nature of the disease. Sometimes the sufferer can talk normally, and on other occasions he can hardly be heard, or produces rapid incomprehensible mumblings. Often he is accused of not trying.

For too long the speech therapist was rarely invited to treat such patients, and often her attitude itself did little to improve the situation. Fortunately this is changing, and the speech therapist's aim to enable the patient to retain independence, and maximize its use of residual communicative skills, involves her actively in counselling both patient and carer and in communicating the need for the intervention to other professionals.

ASSESSMENT

Despite the clear need for objective assessment to determine motor speech impairment, there is a lack of standardized procedures available to speech therapists for assessment and the regular monitoring of the effectiveness of therapy that would ensure that treatment is relevant and effective (Young, 1988).

In the past therapists have relied upon perceptual rating scales (Thompson, 1978). Scales specific to the prosodic abnormality have been found to be reliable (Scott and Caird, 1981; Laver, 1981), and their clinical applicability documented (Scott, Caird and Williams, 1985), but in general therapists rely on dysarthria assessments such as the Frenchay assessment (Enderby, 1980) and the Dysarthria Profile (Robertson, 1982), both of which have standardized scoring systems. The use of sound level meters, glottal frequency analysers, and computerized voice analysers cannot be too highly recommended, but often their expense means that they are only available for research purposes, and then only in addition to the standardized assessments mentioned. More normative data using such apparatus is needed before their expense can be justified in routine clinical use. The ideal assessment will probably use both types of method.

TREATMENT METHODS

Speech therapy for degenerative disorders has traditionally been discouraged (Peacher, 1949). Many considered it to be unrealistic, or a life-long obligation (Allan, 1970). Advances in drug management have greatly altered the life expectancy and quality of PD patients and therapy can now aim to maintain communication ability (Young, 1988). Early treatment may retard the inevitable degeneration of communicative function in more slowly progressing neuromuscular disorders (Darley, Aronson and Brown, 1975).

The best results are agreed to occur in patients who are medically stable and where the response to drug therapy has had an effect on speech (Calne, 1970). Scott *et al.* (1983) recommend that therapy is appropriate for many cases, but that referral for assessment should be made as early as possible in all cases (see p. 6).

Prosodic therapy has been well documented and is strongly recommended (Scott *et al.*, 1985). Visual feedback devices such as the Vocalite, Visispeech, Glottal Frequency Analyser, and computerized monitoring, in conjunction with therapy allow the patient to monitor changes in rate, intensity and intonation. They allow the therapist to compare patterns and facilitate objective measurement (Caligiuri and Murray, 1983; Scott and Caird, 1981, 1983; Robertson, 1988). Hanson and Metter (1980) noted that the use of Delayed Auditory Feedback (DAF) reduces rate and increases intelligibility, not only improves speech rate but increases vocal intensity. They later noted that the use of DAF increased physiological speech effort, thereby increasing intensity. Articulatory contacts were stronger in consonant production, thus increasing speaking effort.

It it important to consider that the loss of prosodic features not only results in dull and monotonous speech but also gives the listener the impression that the sufferer is unlikeable, cold, unfeeling, apathetic, or even demented. The sufferer's inability to discriminate between the different prosodic forms does little to help him. Therapy must therefore include exercises emphasizing the retraining of these skills, if it is to be of any value.

Suggestions for facilitation

Facial expression

The facial muscles will respond to icing. The use of strong smelling substances such as onion or a weak solution of ammonia soaked into a cotton wool ball will cause rapid movement of the facial musculature. The use of cartoons and a mirror to match facial expressions can be helpful, as can resistance exercises.

Respiration

The use of pursed lip breathing techniques, is particularly beneficial; generally there is an increase in vocal intensity and respiratory volume.

Voicing

Asking the patient to reverse count can induce voicing. Sucking on an ice cube, or lemon flavoured ice may also facilitate voicing (Scott, Caird and Williams, 1985; McNiven, 1989).

Many other new forms of therapy are being considered for PD patients, but there is a dearth of documentation regarding their application. One method recently attempted and reported is Music Therapy (Crozier and Hamill, 1988). Established music therapy techniques apply these instrumental and vocal exercises and result in gains in phonation, resonance and rhythm. The classes emphasized relaxation, and the sessions resulted in a very positive~response from the sufferers and their relatives. As a group technique it is certainly worthy of further investigation.

In some cases the intelligibility of speech becomes poorer with daily drug fluctuations, and many sufferers are capable of little voicing. For these and more severely handicapped patients, total communication assessment is necessary, and for many the use of communication aids can offer relief from frustration at non-communication, and so increase their social opportunities.

The introduction of alphabet systems has improved the patient's overall communicative ability (Chen, 1971). Fawcus *et al.* (1983) stress the need for all severely speech handicapped sufferers to have access to a communication board. The only requirements are an ability to select and spell on the part of the sufferer and understanding on the part of the listener. Several electronic aids are now available; all patients and therapists are able to contact communication aid centres throughout Britain for advice and assessment for the most appropriate aid.

Studies of the use made of these centres would indicate that most PD patients are referred for writing aids such as electronic typewriters or Litewriters. It is important to remember that these and other communication aids are not the last resort that many regard them; rather they open up new and better communication channels (Scott, J., personal communication).

96

Traditional methods of therapy are still appropriate for many patients. These are summarized in Scott, Caird and Williams (1985). Today however there are many updated therapy options, and some have been proved to benefit PD sufferers considerably (Scott *et al.*, 1981, 1983; Robertson and Thomson, 1984).

Speech amplification (Greene and Watson, 1968) is considered beneficial in relieving anxiety for those with inaudible speech, whose intelligibility of speech is otherwise intact. The aid reduces tension and by facilitating relaxation, it may reduce tremor, rigidity and akinesia. The amplification of too quiet speech results in the patient matching the amplified output. Green (1980) argues that patients automatically match this level for some time after the aid has been switched off. This gives a considerable psychological boost to the patient, which in turn reinforces a louder level of voice. It is a particularly useful aid if spouse or carer has a hearing loss. It is not indicated when there are other factors influencing speech; it does depend on the sufferer being willing to carry such an aid around with him.

Group therapy (Robertson and Young, 1984) has been found to be a most effective form of intensive therapy. During the two weeks therapy period patients undergo training in techniques designed to improve respiratory control and capacity, vocal coordination, pitch variation, articulatory accuracy, agility and control, and the control of respiratory rate and volume for correct vocal production. This form of therapy has been adopted by many therapist and is well received by sufferers. Group treatment has also become a part of the holiday settings supplied by the Parkinson's Disease Society (Smith *et al.*, 1984; Smith *et al.*, 1985). The Scottish holidays have been joint concerns of physiotherapy and speech therapy; the results of such ventures have been most encouraging. An interesting feature of this type of intervention is the use of recreational hydrotherapy. This is a means of exercising patients in a warm-water gravity-free environment. It facilitates relaxation and as a consequence increases mobility. The acoustic environment and the increased relaxation, also heighten the vocal output in some cases resulting in spontaneous and loud singing!

Simple physical exercises performed in the water with the patients supported by flotation aids, incorporated both vocal and physical rhythms. The reaction of the sufferers was most encouraging. For many it was the first time in the water since childhood and the feelings of freedom and relaxation were greatly appreciated. Patients were highly motivated and responded well to the instant improvement. This is a form of therapy that requires further study as a possible therapy tool (McNiven, 1989). There are contra-indications: severe physical immobility associated with incontinence, epilepsy, heart disease, and skin disease. The speech therapist should work with a physiotherapist at all times and the therapists should be competent in poolside life-saving techniques. All normal precautions associated with the more elderly, disabled person should be taken.

There is still little information regarding the efficacy of dysarthria therapy in general, but it is encouraging that much of what is reported pertains to the treatment of PD patients. With many new possibilities for further study it would seem that speech therapists already have much of value to offer these patients, and much to gain professionally. The progressive and changing nature of PD means that regular review is necessary. Short periods of intensive therapy followed by six monthly assessments are to be seen as positive treatment (Young, 1989). Slowly interest within the speech therapy profession is gaining momentum, it is hoped that this will be matched by an interest from the medical profession.

The Parkinson's Disease Society is one of the most forward-looking charitable organizations in Britain today. Its speech therapy working party exists to offer advice to their own profession and to the membership of the society. Study days have taken place throughout Britain, for speech therapists, doctors, related medical care staffs and more recently specific days for relatives and carers. The working party has produced a Speech Therapy Information Pack for use clinically and current work includes a joint therapy venture to produce a Carers Handbook.

Proven assessment and therapeutic techniques thus exist for the care of PD patients. It is to be hoped that there will be a more positive attitude towards their use by speech therapists, and an increase in the referrals made to speech therapy departments generally.

THE PARKINSONIAN SWALLOWING DISORDER

Swallowing problems are common in PD (Robbins *et al.*, 1985), may occur in as many as 50% of sufferers, and may occasionally be the presenting feature (Croxson, 1988). Though they may be unrelated to the severity of the disease, they tend to increase as the disease progresses. They may be of nuisance value only or may be severe, when they are usually most distressing to the sufferer and carer alike and can cause much social isolation. Many families withdraw from social activities, dread eating out, and avoid such occasions wherever possible. Sufferers may choose to eat alone or may be encouraged to eat at different times from the family to avoid the distressing results of drooling, poor hand to mouth control and the resulting messy eating habits.

It is important to assess the problem as fully and as soon as possible, because PD patients are at risk of silent aspiration from their disordered swallowing, their reduced awareness, and their reduced cough reflex (Robbins et al., 1985).

Dysphagia may be attributed to several factors: the effects of rigidity result in an inadequate range of intraoral muscle function and poor bolus formation and control; poor or abnormal oral and pharyngeal motility results from the same inadequate muscle function and a lack of sensation, from the lack of stimulation of the posterior tongue by the bolus; there are abnormal responses to oropharyngeal somatosensory stimuli (Robbins et al., 1985). It is important to listen to patients' reports of their particular difficulty in swallowing, as they are often very accurate in pinpointing the nature of the problem. They may deny there is a swallowing problem, because failure to recognize difficulties and loss of concentration may lead to a lack of appreciation that meal times are prolonged. A slow eating time may result from rapidly repeated tongue pumping action and consequent delay in transit. Some drugs cause dryness of the mouth (see above) and loss of appetite. Pocketing of food results from lack of buccal tone. Initiation difficulties and swallowing rehearsals are common. These piecemeal movements hinder an adequate swallow, diminish stimulation, cause lack of concentration, fatigue the patient, and may cause aspiration. A delayed swallowing reflex may result from lack of awareness of the stimulation needed to trigger the swallowing response. Laryngeal closure may become inadequate.

Swallowing assessment is usually done by observation by the therapist at the bedside. This relies heavily on the therapist's experience and expertise, and should take up to 45 minutes for a thorough examination (Splaingard et al., 1988), but even a subjective bedside assessment can reveal the following problems: pocketing of food, lengthy eating times, excessive lingual movements (felt under the mandible during chewing), a gurgly voice, and choking during swallowing. The assessment can pinpoint some oral problems but the possibility of pharyngeal difficulties can only be inferred, and the possibility of aspiration is clearly underestimated.

Videofluoroscopic analysis is very useful in a dynamic process (Robbins *et al.*, 1985; Scott, 1988). It allows analysis of the various anatomical structures involved and enables assessment of the shape and position of the bolus. It is neither time-consuming nor invasive and though it could be argued that it is expensive and that it exposes the patient to radiation, it permits early identification of problems, alerts the therapist to the possibility of aspiration, and allows prompt treatment to prevent pneumonia. The ideal assessment thus uses videofluoroscopy. In some cases the technique allows the patient to see himself swallowing and thus heighten his awareness of it. It can illustrate to relatives and carers that despite the lengthy and apparently ineffective action of eating, the patient is in fact making maximum efforts; for many this can relieve misunderstanding and tension. Because it can identify silent aspiration, it is highly recommended when it is available.

TREATMENT OF SWALLOWING PROBLEMS

The swallowing difficulties may respond to levodopa (Bushmann *et al.*, 1989). However, they will not necessarily resolve together with the general Parkinsonian symptoms. In some cases the response is minimal and swallowing is worse with medication. It is imperative that all PD sufferers are assessed for dysphagic difficulties since they are in danger of silent aspiration. Although the more serious problems are associated with the later stages of the disease, aspiration and vallecular pocketing may occur early in some cases.

The primary aim is to establish a safe and functional swallow. Ideally the patient should be treated in a comfortable position, in an appropriate chair, not a wheelchair. If the patient has to be treated in bed, the same degree of comfort is necessary; he should be well supported by pillows, his head should be in the midline, and his neck muscles neither flexed nor extended.

If there is any possibility of aspiration, the therapist should always work with someone competent in suction techniques.

Some speech therapists may be confident and competent to carry out oral and pharyngeal suction, but the patient's comfort and safety demand that no form of suction should be attempted by someone not well rehearsed in the technique.

The therapist must consider all factors that may affect swallowing and eating. The fit and functional use of the patient's dentures should be assessed first. Many PD patients complain of ill-fitting dentures, which are uncomfortable and unsightly, and further handicap speech. A thin metallic upper denture plate, rather than the usual acrylic one, increases intraoral feedback, and is more easily retained, and better tolerated by the weaker oral musculature. Building up the lower buccal sulcus (Selley and Tudor, 1974) – a common dental aid in stroke patients – may also be beneficial in PD patients. The increased bulk along the lower gum ridge gives the muscles a better grip, and may improve retention.

Patients at home or in wards for the elderly may have other factors affecting their swallowing. There may be physical problems in handling cutlery and transferring food from the plate to the mouth, which are best assessed by the occupational therapist (p. 83), though the speech therapist should be aware of what is available to help in such cases.

When all the other factors have been considered, the speech therapist can attempt to alleviate the swallowing problems present. In an extremely ill patient the therapist is trying to elicit a swallowing reflex, and some of the following exercises may help. However most patients are referred because of mild or moderate problems, and then the therapist is attempting to improve tongue and lip function, improve the swallowing pattern, and heighten the patient's awareness of the swallowing process.

Treatment suggestions

Lip control

The use of a lip sensor device in conjunction with a mirror can improve poor lip posture and control, thereby alleviating drooling. The use of taste can also improve the effectiveness of therapy. Flavouring the ice cubes with citric tastes, or salty/sweet tastes may help. It is important to remember, since not all flavours are liked by everyone, to ask the patient what flavours he prefers. Having flavoured the ice, apply the cube centrally. The patient has to suck on the cube. Applying the cube to the under surface of the top lip and moving between the gum ridge and top teeth causes rapid lip closure. Dropping small amounts of sherry or lime juice from a syringe or pipette onto closed lips will cause tongue tip protrusion and a swallow. It is important that this is done working in front of the patient, giving visual and verbal stimulation concurrently with the icing. Try to stand in view but to the side of the mirror in order that the patient gets maximum feedback.

Tongue control

Ice to the lower lip facilitates tip protrusion and in some cases a reflex swallow. Ice applied to the sides of the lips encourages tongue movement from side to side. Jabbing the tongue tip with a spatula rapidly, causes tip protrusion and pulling gently on the tongue tip can result in retraction. The resistance exercises of Langley and Darvill (1979) are also most beneficial.

Palatal control

Over and above the normal blowing and sucking exercises, the use of quinine or angostura bitters on a cotton wool bud, applied to the back of the tongue and the velum can produce the desired response.

Mastication

Soft cheese or soft cheddar, ham or smoked fish flavours, chewed on the back molars can increase the chewing action and increase masticatory strength.

It is important to consider the types and flavours of foods that the patient might try. A dietician can recommend many excellent suggestions, and the diet sheet provided by the Parkinson's Disease Society Speech Therapy Information pack is strongly recommended.

REFERENCES

Allan, C.M. (1970) Treatment of non-fluent speech resulting from neurological diseases – treatment of dysarthria. *British Journal of Disorders of Communication*, **5**, 1–4.

Bushmann, M., Dobmeyer, S.M., Leeker, L. and Perlmutter, J.S. (1989) Swallowing abnormalities and their response to treatment in Parkinson's disease. *Neurology*, **39**, 1309–14.

Butfield, C. (1961) Dysarthria, Speech Pathology and Therapy, **4**, 74.

Calne, D.B. (1970) *Parkinsonism: Physiology, Pharmacology and Treatment*. Edward Arnold, London.

Canter, G.J. (1963) Speech characteristics of patients with Parkinson's disease: I Intensity, patch and duration. *Journal of Speech and Hearing Disorders*, **28**, 221–29.

Canter, G.J. (1965a) Speech characteristics of patients with Parkinson's disease: II Physiological support for speech. *Journal of Speech and Hearing Disorders*, **30**, 44–9.

Canter, G.J. (1965b) Speech characteristics of patients with Parkinson's disease: III Articulation, diadochokinesis and overall speech adequacy. *Journal of Speech and Hearing Disorders*, **30**, 217–23.

Caligiuiri, M.P. and Murry, T. (1983) The use of visual feedback to enhance prosodic control in dysarthria. *Clinical Dysarthria*, Berry, W. (ed.). College-Hill Press, San Diego.

Chen, L.Y. (1971) Manual communication by combined alphabet and gesture. *Archives of Physical Medical Rehabilitation*, **52**, 381–84.

Critchley, E.M.R. (1981) Speech disorders of Parkinsonism: A review. *Journal of Neurology and Neurosurgery and Psychiatry*, **44**, 751–58.

Croxson, S.C.M. (1988) Dysphagia as the presenting feature of Parkinson's disease. *Geriatric Medicine*, **18**, 16.

Crozier, E. and Hamill, R. (1988) The benefits of combining speech and music therapy. *Speech Therapy in Practice*, **4**, 18.

Darley, G.L., Aronson, A.E. and Brown, J.R. (1975) *Motor Speech Disorders*. W.B. Saunders, Philadelphia.

Enderby, P. (1980) *The Frenchay Dysarthria Assessment*. College-Hill Press, San Diego.

Fawcus, M., Williams, R., Williams, J. and Robinson, M. (eds) (1983) *Working with Dysphasics*. Winslow Press Ltd., Winslow, Buckinghamshire.

Gawel, M.J. (1981) The effects of various drugs on speech. *British Journal of Disorders of Communication*, **16**, 51–7.

Gotham, A.M., Brown, R.G. and Marsden, C.D. (1986) Depression and Parkinson's disease: a qualitative and quantitative analysis. *Journal of Neurology, Neurosurgery and Psychiatry*, **49**, 381–9.

Greene, M.C.L. (1980) *The Voice and its Disorders*, 4th ed. 306–16. Pitman, London.

Greene, M.C.L. and Watson, B.W. (1968) The value of speech amplification in Parkinson's disease. *Folia Phoniatrica*, **20**, 250–7.

Hanson, W.R. and Metter, E.J. (1980) DAF as an instrumental treatment for dysarthria in supranuclear palsy: A case report. *Journal of Speech and Hearing Disorders*, **45**, 268–76.

Hutchinson, J.M. and Beasley, D.S. (1976) Speech and language functioning among the ageing, in *Ageing and Communication* (eds H.J. Oyer and E.J. Oyer) University Park Press, Baltimore.

Johnson, J.A. (1988) An in depth Assessment of Short Course Speech Therapy in Parkinsonian Patients. MSc. Thesis. The City University.

Judge, T.J. and Caird, F.I. (1977) *Drug Treatment of the Elderly Patient*. Pitman Medical, Tunbridge Wells.

Kammermeier, M.A. (1969) *A Comparison of Phonatory Phenomena among Groups of Neurologically Impaired Speakers*. Ph.D. Dissertation. University of Minnesota.

Kim, R. (1968) The chronic residual respiratory disorder in post-encephalitic Parkinsonism. *Journal of Neurology and Neurosurgery and Psychiatry*, **31**, 393–98.

Langley, J. and Darvill, G. 1979) *Procedures for Facilitating Improvements in Swallow, Mastication, Speech and Facial Expression where these have been impaired by Central or Peripheral Nerve Damage*. College of Speech Therapists. London.

Laver, J. (1981) *Phonetic Description of Voice Quality*. Cambridge University Press, Cambridge.

McNiven, D.R. (1989) *Swallowing Facilitation*. College of Speech Therapists Advanced Course: Care of the Elderly, Glasgow.

Marsden, C.D. and Parkes, J.D. (1976) 'On-off' effects on patients with Parkinson's disease on chronic levodopa therapy. *Lancet*, **1**, 292–6.

Mawdsley, C. and Gamsu, C.V. (1971) Periodicity of speech in Parkinsonism. *Nature*, **23**, 865–70.

Mueller, P.B. (1971) Parkinson's disease: Motor speech behaviour in a selected group of patients. *Folia Phoniatrica*, **23**, 333–46.

Mutch, W.J., Strudwick, A., Roy, S.K. and Downie, A.W. (1986) Parkinson's disease: disability, review and management. *British Medical Journal*, **293**, 675–77.

Nakano, K.K., Zubick, H. and Tyler, H.R. (1973) Speech defect of Parkinsonian patients: effect of levodopa therapy on speech intelligibility. *Neurology*, **23**, 865–970.

Oxtoby, M. (982) *Parkinson's Disease Patients and their Social Needs*, Parkinson's Disease Society, London.

Parkes, J.C. (1982) *Parkinson's Disease*. Updated Postgraduate Series. Update Publications Ltd, London.

Peacher, W.G. (1949) Etiology and differential diagnosis of dysarthria. *Journal of Speech and Hearing Disorders*, **15**, 252–65.

Ptacek, P.H., Sander, E.K., Moloney, W.H. and Jackson, C. (1966)

Phonatory and related changes with advanced age. *Journal of Speech and Hearing Research*, **9**, 353–60.

Rigrodsky, S. and Morrison, E. (1970) Speech changes in Parkinsonism during L-dopa therapy: preliminary findings. *Journal of the American Geriatric Society*, **18**, 142–51.

Robbins, J.A., Logemann, J.A., and Kirschner, H.S. (1985). Swallowing and speech production in Parkinson's disease. *Annals of Neurology*, **19**, 283–87.

Robertson, S.J. (1982) *The Dysarthria Profile*. London.

Robertson, S.J. (1988) Parkinson's disease: Does speech therapy work, and defining the problems. *Speech Therapy in Practice*, **4**, 18–19.

Robertson, S.J. and Thomson, F. (1984) Speech therapy in Parkinson's disease: a study of the efficacy and long term effects of intensive treatment. *British Journal of Disorders of Communication*, **19**, 213–24.

Ryan, W.J. and Burke, K.W. (1974) Perceptual and acoustic correlates of ageing in the speech of males. *Journal of Disorders of Communication*, **7**, 181.

Scott, S. and Caird, F.I. (1981) Speech therapy for patients with Parkinson's disease. *British Medical Journal*, **283**, 1088.

Scott, S., Caird, F.I. and Williams, B.O. (1983) Speech therapy for Parkinson's disease. *Journal of Neurology, Neurosurgery and Psychiatry*, **46**, 140–44.

Scott, S. and Caird, F.I. (1984) The response of the apparent receptive speech disorder of Parkinson's disease to speech therapy. *Journal of Neurology, Neurosurgery and Psychiatry*, **47**, 302–4.

Scott, S., Caird, F.I. and Williams, B.O. (1985) *Communication in Parkinson's disease*. Croom Helm, Kent.

Scott, S. (1988) Parkinson's disease: Treatment can reduce social isolation. *Speech Therapy in Practice*, **4**, 21.

Selley, W.G. and Tudor, C. (1974) A palatal training appliance and visual aid for use in the treatment of hypernasal speech. *British Journal of Disorders of Communication*, **9**, 117–22.

Smith, R.G., Bowman, I., McNiven, D.R. and Scott, S. (1984) *Therapeutic Holiday*. Edinburgh University Department of Geriatric Medicine (unpublished).

Smith, R.G. (1985) Therapeutic Holiday: Report on the Parkinson's Disease Society Holiday, 1983. *Edinburgh Medicine*, April.

Splaingard, M.L., Hutchins, B., Sulton, L.D. and Chaudhuri, G. (1988) Aspiration in rehabilitation patients: video-fluoroscopy *vs* bedside clinical examination. *Archives of Physical Medical and Rehabilitation*, **69**, 637–40.

Thompson, A.K. (1978) A clinical rating scale for speech dysfunction in Parkinson's disease. *South African Journal of Communication Disorders*, **25** 39–52.

Uziel, A., Bohe, M., Cadilhac, J. and Passouant, P. (1975) Les troubles de la voix et de la parole dans les syndromes Parkinsoniens. *Folia Phoniatrica*, **27**, 166–76.

Young, F. (1988) *Speech Therapy in Practice*, Parkinson's disease: management strategies, **4**, 19.

Young, F. (1989) *Treatment in PD*. Study Day Lecture. Stoke Mandeville Hospital.

Weismer, G. (1984) Articulatory characteristics of Parkinsonian dysarthria: segmental and phrase level timing, spiratization and glottal supraglottal coordination. In *The Dysarthrias: Physiology, Acoustics, and Management*. McNeil, M.R., Rosenbek, J.C., Aronson, A.E., (eds). College-Hill Press, San Diego.

7

The social worker

Mary Baker and Pauline Smith

Acquiring knowledge about Parkinson's disease involves absorbing impersonal and objective facts: facts about incidence and mean ages, about the basal ganglia, the substantia nigra, neurotransmitters and chemical actions and reactions. This information, and much more can be found in other chapters of this book, and in other text-books on the subject. However, Parkinson's disease affects people: men and women from different age groups, different races and cultures, and different social backgrounds. What this chapter is concerned with, and what the social worker's professional skills have the expertise to discern, is an understanding and an awareness of the implications of Parkinson's disease for those who live with it.

Understanding and awareness involve feeling and empathy, and are best achieved by listening and talking to the people who have the condition, and to the husbands, wives, other relatives or friends, who care for them daily, and nightly, in their homes. It is only through understanding and awareness that the social worker will be able to abstract from the common facts of PD and focus on the particular and personal needs for the people who live with it.

UNDERSTANDING PARKINSON'S DISEASE

PD can be defined as a disorder of movement which affects learned, voluntary actions. But what does this mean to the people who have the condition and those who care for them? Consider the activities involving learned, voluntary actions which people perform everyday, and which make life not only possible but worthwhile. The following list is by no means comprehensive:

Walking, eating, washing, getting out of bed, talking, cooking, household chores, going to the toilet, dressing, climbing stairs, shopping, bathing, cleaning teeth, answering the telephone, turning over in bed, gardening, sport, driving, using public transport, working, writing, dancing, sex, going out, rising from a chair, playing musical instruments, hobbies, body language, socializing.

PD therefore can, to some degree, affect every aspect of life. No two people will experience exactly the same difficulties or the same level of difficulty, but the social worker should be constantly aware of real and potential problems facing individuals and families, and of the consequences these will have.

Grouping some of these activities together makes the implications apparent: difficulties with mobility and dexterity affect working, driving, using public transport, walking, getting out of bed, rising from a chair, hobbies, household chores, gardening, going out, and socializing. The implications for both the person with PD and the carer include financial problems, role reversal, isolation, bordom, frustration, and depression. The person with PD will experience loss of independence and self-esteem, and the carer feelings of being depended upon, lack of freedom, and tiredness.

Difficulties with communication include problems with talking, writing, using the telephone, and body language (including posture, gesture, and facial expression), and the implications for both the person with PD and the carer are withdrawal, isolation, frustration, depression, loss of companionship, and breakdown in relationships.

Difficulties associated with personal care, with washing, cleaning the teeth, dressing, eating, bathing, going to the toilet, turning in bed, produce resentment and anger in both patient and carer, loss of dignity and privacy, embarrassment and frustration in the patient, and tiredness and lack of sleep in the carer.

Treatment of PD involves the use of drug therapy which will need to be tailored to the individual's needs by the neurologist or geriatrician, and reviewed regularly by the general practitioner. Many of the more effective anti-Parkinsonian drugs have unwanted side-effects which vary in type and severity from one person to another, and will grow more apparent as treatment continues. Sufficient information should be given to the person with PD and the carer so that they can recognize side effects and distinguish them from the symptoms of the condition itself. The general practitioner or hospital consultant will be the best person with whom to discuss this. It is also important to be aware that people with PD will suffer from other ailments which should be treated independently of the PD, and should not be assumed to be integral and unavoidable symptoms of the condition or side effects of the drugs involved.

There are certain features of PD which require further explanation. They need sympathetic and careful handling and the social worker will need to ensure that all the people involved in care and support understand them and deal appropriately with them.

Freezing (p. 5) episodes last a variable time. Many sufferers devise their own 'tricks' to help regain mobility, so it is worthwhile asking them or their carers what help is needed. The 'on-off' syndrome (p. 5) is also a sudden change in ability, but unlike freezing which is a symptom of PD, is an adverse effect of long-term levodopa therapy. Patients first experiencing 'on–off' may want to take their drugs more frequently, but this is not necessarily the best course of action, and medical referral for guidance on drug therapy is essential. Both freezing and the 'on-off' pheonomenon can be very frustrating for the person with PD and the carer.

Even from a professional carer's point of veiw it may seem that the person is being deliberately obstructive and uncooperative, since at certain times of the day they are mobile and able to cope well, whilst at others they appear to be making no effort at all. It takes a great deal of understanding, both of the condition and of the needs of individual people to recognize 'on-off' and to deal sympathetically with it.

In addition to the rapid switch of 'on–off' many people with Parkinson's disease experience 'good' times, 'bad' times and even 'good' days and 'bad' days, and will need to arrange their activities as best they can around these times (p. 70).

Abnormal involuntary movements are associated with long-term treatment of levodopa. As with all other aspects of Parkinson's disease they will vary in type and severity from one person to another. The restless movements of the hands or feet, or uncontrollable writhing of the whole body are in complete contrast to the immobility experienced at other times of the day. They may be distressing and embarrassing to the person with PD and the carer, or they may provide the energy and mobility required to perform everyday tasks. Some involuntary movement therefore may be preferable to no movement at all. The feelings of each individual need to be taken into account by the consultant when re-assessing and balancing drug therapy, so that the maximum benefits, and the minimum unwanted side-effects are achieved.

THE MANAGEMENT OF PARKINSON'S DISEASE

PD affects each individual differently with regard to symptoms, progress of the disease, and response to the benefits and side-effects of drug therapy. Careful, individual management therefore is the key to improving and maintaining quality of life for both the patient and the carer, and this is best achieved by a multidisciplinary team approach. Ideally, all the members of the team will be involved as soon as possible following diagnosis (p. 111). In this way assessment and re-assessment of need will continue, and treatment, advice and support will be modified as the condition progresses and individual responses and circumstances change. Ideally the patient and the carer will be involved in decisions concerning treatment and care, and their experiences and expertise will be acknowledged and valued.

Referral to the social worker and the therapists often only occurs when the carer can no longer cope, when speech is no longer intelligible, when mobility has ceased, or when independent living is no longer a possibilty. Yet early referral will enable relationships of confidence and trust to be established, assessment, advice and appropriate action to be taken which will alleviate, or at the very least postpone, the breakdown in relationships, the loss and the distress associated with crisis management. Oxtoby (1982) found that 54% of people with Parkinson's disease had never had a visit from a social worker.

The majority of people with PD live in their own homes; 17% of these live alone, and 50% live with partners who themselves suffer from illness or disability (Oxtoby, 1982). It is important therefore for the social worker to visit the home at the earliest opportunity to assess the family relationships and establish whether family care networks exist in reality. The carer's physical and psychological health is of the utmost importance. It is only by seeing people within their own environment, listening to them, giving them time, and utilizing skills of observation and perception, that the social worker will be able to judge where help is necessary and what referrals need to be made.

At diagnosis

The social worker will need listening and counselling skills to explore the feelings and levels of understanding of the person with PD and the carer, and should be aware of a number of factors which will influence the way the diagnosis is received. Peoples' perceptions of illness and disability will be influenced by their social and cultural backgrounds, their age, and their prior experiences, understanding, or misunderstanding of a particular condition. Thus the diagnosis of PD may be received with feelings of horror and fear, isolation, guilt, anger and injustice. Early symptoms are often non-specific, and diagnosis is therefore sometimes problematic. Tests and referrals to eliminate other conditions may take time during which people will have had their own thoughts, and fears, about what may be wrong with them. Being given a 'label' – a medical term which gives credence to the way they feel – and the offer of therapy to relieve their symptoms, may therefore be greeted with great relief. However, sometimes, feelings of relief quickly give way to anxieties about the future, and the effect that the condition will have on personal and social relationships, and the ability to maintain an independent and worthwhile life. Younger Parkinsonians – one in seven are diagnosed under the age of 50 – may have believed that the condition only affects the elderly, and may refuse to accept the diagnosis or discuss it with partners, children, or colleagues. It is important for people to be given the opportunity to examine their fears and feelings to know that these are normal, natural reactions to the news they have been given, and to understand that they are not alone.

Information concerning the Parkinson's Disease Soicety, the local branch, and the Younger Parkinsonian's group should be made available so that if they want to they can contact other people who understand and live with the condition. A wealth of knowledge, understanding, friendship and support can be found within the branches of the Society and the Younger Parkinsonian's group. Literature about PD and information concerning the help, advice, and support that is available from the different members of the multidisciplinary team is also important. Reassurance should be given about the diversity of symptoms, and that no two people experience the same problems. People should be encouraged to remain as active as possible and to continue with their daily routines, adjusting and substituting other activities only when the need arises.

A further factor which influences the way people feel when they hear that they or their partner have PD, is the way that they are told by the hospital specialist and the information which is given to them at the time. Ideally, after giving the diagnosis, and establishing the patient's prior knowledge and understanding of PD, the doctor will give a short but honest and positive explanation of the condition and the appropriate drug therapy. People are unable to assimilate detailed, complex information at this time and yet they will want to understand what is happening to them and why, how it will affect their lives, and what can be done to help them. It is only after they have had the opportunity to come to terms with the news, and reflect on the implications of it, that they will be ready for more detailed explanations. They will then be able to ask pertinent and meaningful questions, and be sufficiently informed to make choices and decisions concerning their future. Literature giving information and advice can be obtained from the Parkinson's Disease Society.

Following the commencement of drug therapy, the majority of people respond well. Some even claim a 'miracle cure', or that the diagnosis must have been wrong and that they do not have PD at all. False hopes may need to be confronted to avoid severe disappointments later. This period is often referred to as the 'honeymoon period' when the benefits of the drugs far outweigh any side-effects which may occur. Nevertheless the condition will continue to progress and new symptoms will emerge from time-to-time.

When the 'honeymoon' is over

Depression and sudden mood changes are common features of PD. Quite natural feelings of sadness, lack of motivation and irritability due to increasing awareness of loss and dependency, or severe depression and even suicidal tendencies which appear to outweigh the degree of physical disability. Hallucinations and frightening nightmares are known side-effects of levodopa therapy and the possibility of drug-induced psychosis should not be ignored. Counselling, adjustments to drug therapy, and the introduction of anti-depressant drugs may all be beneficial. The social worker will need to be aware of the significance of mood changes and depression in PD and, in consultation with the general practitioner, assess whether referral to the consultant, a psychiatrist, psychiatric social worker, or community psychiatric nurse are appropriate.

Depression in carers is also common. Caring full-time for someone with a progressive physical disability is in itself physically and emotionally exhausting, but caring from someone who is also suffering from depression and sudden inexplicable mood swings causes further distress. 'I can cope with doing all the extra things – but it's the companionship I miss. I don't know him any more – it's like living with a stranger'. Carers often feel trapped in their new and unwelcome role because of family, cultural or social expectations and their own feelings of duty. Some carers are sustained by their love and their memories of a fulfilled and happy relationship, but others will not be able to draw on such benefits. The social worker should take time to explore the present and past relationship between the couple, and help the carer work through natural feelings of anger and resentment, and examine common feelings of guilt. The Carer's National Association provides information, advice and counselling, and a local carer's group will provide a forum for sharing support and companionship.

As the condition progresses

It is now recognized that pain is a feature of PD, and may occur particularly at night in conjunction with leg or arm cramps. Sometimes the pain and cramping is so severe that the patient is unable to sleep. Painkillers may be of some help and advice should be sought from the general practitioner or consultant. Being aware of the possible severity of pain, professional carers will be better equipped to understand and manage the distress and the restlessness it causes.

Turning over in bed is a particular problem for people with PD, and they may need to wake the carer, or call for help from the nurse or care attendant if they are unable to turn themselves. Toileting may become a real trial, partly because of the rigidity and immobility, and partly because of the inability to initiate micturition once at the toilet or when given a bottle or bedpan. There is a need to urinate but no result. This can be very frustrating for the person concerned and those caring for them, especially if it happens several times a night, and it requires considerable understanding and patience to avoid distress.

Facial expression and body language form a very important part of communication. Unfortunately rigidity deprives people with PD of this form of expression and subtle communication (p. 93). Constant care should be taken to avoid assumptions that people with PD are unresponsive, bored, or unintelligent, and initial feelings of dislike should be examined and reasoned. Pentland *et al.* (1987) questioned the effects that loss of body language can have on therapeutic relationships and the patient's self-image, concluding that there was a need for 'all health professionals to take account of their first impressions of Parkinsonian patients, to consider the role non-verbal signals have had in their formulation and to guard against overhasty assumptions about mood, personality and intellect.' These recommendations are equally relevant to social workers, home helps or care attendants in residential homes.

Difficulties in initiating thoughts, speech, and actions, and the physical and psychological stress involved in caring will increase as the condition progresses. The person with PD and the caring partner may themselves be unable to realize their needs or be aware of the local services to which they are entitled. The social worker will require great sensitivity in identifying the needs of the family and enlisting the help of community services. For example, is the occupational therapist involved in assessing the suitability of the accommodation and are adaptations, equipment and aids needed? Are the services of the home care team, and meals-on-wheels being utilized? Is there a local sitting service which would enable the carer to have free time? Does the community nurse or a bath nurse visit regularly, and are the services of the continence nurse necessary? Is Crossroads involved? Would the day hospital, day centre or a luncheon club provide a social and therapeutic outing for the person with PD and a valuable break for the carer? What are the individual's/family's transport needs, and are they aware of the Orange Badge Scheme? How are prescriptions being collected, and (for those under 65) is use being made of a season ticket? Is the person with PD, and the carer, receiving dental care, and do they need the services of the optometrist and chiropodist? Counsel and

Care for the Elderly provide a useful fact sheet on the statutory and voluntary services which provide help in the home.

All these services will require the involvement of professional and lay personnel who will be experienced and skilled in their own particular field, but not necessarily in PD. Do they understand about 'freezing' episodes, 'on–off', abnormal involuntary movements, slowness, difficulties with initiation, and communication problems? To avoid distress, frustration and misunderstanding and to maximize the benefits of the services provided, the social worker will need to be sensitive to the developing feelings and relationships between the providers of community care and their clients. Professional literature packs are available from the Parkinson's Disease Society.

FINANCIAL WORRIES

Chronic illness and disability, and caring full-time for a disabled or handicapped relative, involve financial as well as physical and emotional costs. The social worker will be able to advise on entitlements and where necessary help to make applications. A number of benefits and allowances, including income support, attendance allowance, mobility allowance and invalid care allowance may be appropriate; the 'Disability Rights Handbook' gives comprehensive information on current rates and eligibility. Information concerning financial matters can be obtained from the local Citizens Advice Bureau and the Parkinson's Disease Society, which will also be able to advise younger Parkinsonians on taking early retirement, mortgage repayments, etc.

Because of the complex nature of Parkinson's disease many people who are entitled, for example to mobility and attendance allowance, are refused because they are 'on' and mobile when they are assessed. For this reason it would be valuable for the social worker to recommend that the carer completes a diary, noting the changes which occur during the day and drawing attention to the realities of living with PD. For example:

Tuesday night:	Very uncomfortable and upset in the night. Couldn't turn over or get to the bathroom. Woke me four times for help.
Wednesday am:	'Off' until after breakfast. Needed help washing, going to toilet, dressing and

	eating. Couldn't walk alone. 'On' and mobile for two hours. Able to walk and go to the toilet.
Wednesday pm:	Started to slow down just before dinner. Needed help eating which took ages. Sat in the chair for over an hour. Tablets are working. Walked into the garden to see the flowers. Looked at the paper and 'helped' me in the kitchen! 'Off' again. Can't move from the chair. Depressed. Crying, etc.

The social worker can also add comments to the diary and encourage the district nurse, home help, relatives and neighbours to do the same

The Independent Living Fund was set up to help severely disabled people on low incomes to pay for care and services which will help them to continue living independently in their own homes. There are a number of Benevolent Funds which may provide funding for specific needs if statutory funding is inadequate. Information concerning Benevolent Funds can be obtained from the Parkinson's Disease Society and the Counsel and Care for the Elderly fact sheet 'Which Charity?'

HOLIDAYS

Due to financial constraints, immobility and transport difficulties, embarrassment at eating in public places and fear of being misunderstood, the patient and carer may have forgone holidays for a number of years. Nevertheless holidays are extremely beneficial, providing a break from the routine of house-bound isolation so often experienced by disabled people and their carers, allowing for the carer to be waited on and cared for, and providing an opportunity to make new friendships and try out new activities which may be continued when the holiday is over. Holidays are available for individuals and couples, with or without therapies and activities such as music and art. Information on holidays, and advice concerning financial help and transport arrangements can be obtained from the Parkinson's Disease Society. Holidays can also be arranged through Social Services, the Winged Fellowship and Holiday Care.

GOING INTO HOSPITAL

Hospital admission to establish a new drug regime or implement changes in drug therapy may be necessary if the condition deteriorates or the drug side effects becomes severe (p. 109). Some patients and their relatives find it difficult to approach doctors to voice their anxieties and it may be in the social worker, with whom a trusting relationship has already been developed, that such confidences are invested. Patients should be encouraged to enter into a partnership with their consultant in order to find the most appropriate dosage and combination of drugs. It is important to establish that both the patient and the carer have a real understanding of what may be a complicated drug regime.

Going into hospital for conditions not related to PD may present particular difficulties to the patient and carer (p. 109). It is usual on most wards for all drugs to be handed in on admission, and subsequently given out on routine drug rounds. It cannot be stressed too strongly how vital it is to maintain the dose and timing of the drug regime which the consultant and patient have spent considerable time establishing. Wards which specialize in orthopaedics, gynaecology or general surgery may have little experience or understanding of chronic neurological conditions like PD. Staff may be distressed and frustrated by the deterioration of their patient's mobility, but not connect it with what appears to be insignificant changes in drug therapy. They may not be aware of the various features mentioned earlier, which will result in assumptions being made about the patient, resentment and anger, and great distress to the patient and carer. The physiotherapist, speech therapist and dietician will be based in the hospital and should be contacted if difficulties with mobility, communication and swallowing are evident. Supporting the person with PD and the carer through the admission, the social worker will be able to assess feelings and levels of understanding, and act appropriately. Nurses' information packs describing the particular features of PD and emphasizing the need to value the expertise of the patient and the carer are available from the Parkinson's Disease Society.

Consideration should be given to how the carer is visiting the patient, and transport arrangements may be necessary. On discharge, adequate community back-up should be ensured in consultation with the doctor, ward sister or medical social worker.

RESPITE CARE

The possibility of respite care should be considered by the social worker and discussed with the carer before the necessity arises. The carer may be reluctant to let the patient go into short-term care and claim that she alone fully understands the partner's needs and difficulties – 'Nobody can look after him the way I can'. It may be necessary to counsel both the patient and the carer to avoid feelings of guilt, resentment and fear of separation. Sadly there have been times when admission to a geriatric ward or Young Disabled Unit has resulted in unhappiness, confusion, bed sores, and a deterioration in PD symptoms which have continued for several weeks after discharge and have meant the carer refusing the offer of respite care again. The social worker can play a valuable role liaising between the carer and nursing staff, providing literature and advice, and reinforcing the carer's personal expertise about their partner's requirements.

SHELTERED, RESIDENTIAL AND NURSING HOME CARE

Despite careful, individual management by the multidisciplinary team, adaptations to the home and a network of community support, the continuing progression of PD, or the inability of the carer to continue caring may mean that special accommodation will need to be considered. In consultation with the general practitioner, the hospital consultant and the family, decisions can be made regarding the level of care required, and whether sheltered accommodation, a residential home or nursing home is appropriate. The social worker's role in the transitional period will be crucial. Feelings of loss, dependence, guilt and fear will need to be confronted, and the benefits of security, appropriate care and companionship suggested as a counter to leaving the familiar surroundings of home. The careful counselling of the person with PD and the carer or other close relatives will be necessary to ensure that the decision is theirs. Only then should information on all possible options be made available to the family, and time for discussion allowed so that informed choices can be made. Information and advice with regard to eligibility, finances, and placement agencies can be obtained from the Parkinson's Disease Society. Counsel and Care for the Elderly and

Age Concern produce comprehensive fact sheets on special accommodation for elderly people.

Before the final choice is made the family will need to visit and view the accommodation. They may need help in asking pertinent questions concerning accommodation, facilities, staff and supervision. If the patient is moving to a residential or nursing home it will be necessary to determine whether the staff have experience and understanding of PD, and whether speech therapy and physiotherapy is available. However, consideration for the physical needs of people with PD should never diminish the social worker's awareness of the people themselves. Their age, personality, religion, culture or ethnic group may be essential prerequisites to whether they will feel relaxed, happy and welcomed in what is to be their last home. It is also important to find out about visiting arrangements. For instance, will the carer be able to spend time in the home and possibly stay overnight?

The social worker's role will continue in the management of Parkinson's disease even when the final decisions have been agreed and the move has taken place. During the final stages of PD, patients will be at their most frail and vulnerable, yet quality of life, dignity and, as far as possible, independence should still be the objective. The consciousness of the caring staff, concerning the complex and often bizarre nature of PD, will need to be raised, and the medical, social and personal implications of it understood. It should never be forgotten that beneath the 'mask' is a person who needs to be held, touched, loved, praised, encouraged and listened to.

REFERENCES

Oxtoby, M. (1982) *Parkinson's Disease Patients and their Social Needs.* Parkinson's Disease Society, London.

Pentland, B., Pitcairn, T.K. Gray, J.M. and Riddle W.J.R. (1987) The effects of reduced expression in Parkinson's disease on impression formation by health professionals. *Clinical Rehabilitation*, **1**, 307.

8

The Parkinson's Disease Society

Mary Baker and Bridget McCall

The Parkinson's Disease Society was founded in 1969 by Miss Mali Jenkins (1904–1989), whose sister, Sarah, had PD. She was surprised to find that no society existed to help people suffering from PD and their families. From her experience of caring for Sarah, she knew that there was a desperate need for greater public understanding of PD and the problems that it brings, as well as the support that such a society could offer. With the help of her sister Eryl, Mali Jenkins set about founding the society from a bedroom in her house. Initially its aim was to provide an information service, but as the demand grew, the services that the society offered expanded. Since then the society has become a major charity supporting important research into scientific and welfare aspects of PD, as well as promoting mutual self-help for sufferers and their carers through the activities of its 160 branches.

Most of the society's income is derived from voluntary donations, bequests, and fundraising activities initiated both by its head office and its branches. There is a membership scheme, but it is important to stress that the society exists to help all people suffering from PD and their carers; it makes no distinction between members and non-members in terms of the help that it offers.

The society has three aims:

1. To help patients and their relatives with the problems arising from Parkinson's disease.
2. To collect and disseminate information on Parkinson's disease.
3. To encourage and provide funds for research into Parkinson's disease.

Much of the society's work is in three fields – research, welfare and branch development. In addition a great deal of literature is produced to help sufferers and their carers as well as professionals responsible for their care. There is a quarterly newsletter which gives information on activities within the society and a branch bulletin to cover the branch activities. The society is also involved in publicity work to improve the public's awareness of Parkinson's disease and to encourage support.

MEDICAL RESEARCH

In 1988 over £500 000 was spent on medical research (in addition to funds allocated to the brain bank – see below). The society supports nearly thirty medical research projects in establishments throughout the country currently working to find the cause and cure for Parkinson's disease and also to improve current treatments.

The society's brain bank is a special unit, which is investigating the brain and other relevant tissues of sufferers from PD in the hope that this will provide clues that will lead to the cause and cure of the disease. Tissue is donated by sufferers for use after death in a similar way to other organ donation schemes. Certain criteria have to be met for the tissue to be of value to research. The Brain Bank research focuses on processes in the brain which may be involved in PD. Much research is being done into Lewy bodies (p. 3), which have also been shown to occur in the gullet and large intestine.

Since it is thought that PD may be caused by some toxic substance in the environment, much work is being done in the biochemical background to PD, such as iron metabolism and free radicals. Research in other establishments includes studies on MPTP (pp. 2 and 23), which may improve existing chemical models of PD (Truscott, 1988). Motor and cognitive abilities and impairment in PD patients are also being studied, as well as work to improve diagnosis and detect pre-clinical PD using PET scanners.

The society was founded around the time that the deficit of dopamine in the brains of patients with PD was first demonstrated. Much of the work that the society funds is concerned with aspects of drug treatment, for instance, to try to isolate the receptor for dopamine in the brain. It may be that the drugs can

121

be designed to fit the receptor more accurately and thereby be more effective (Strange, 1989). Trials are also being done on other drug therapies such as apomorphine infusion (Pearce, 1989). The society is also supporting the much publicized research by Professor Edward Hitchcock into fetal brain cell implantation into Parkinsonian brains.

The support that the society gives to research is therefore wide-ranging. To promote this valuable work amongst professionals the society has also organized several international symposia on current research into PD.

WELFARE

Oxtoby (1982) carried out a survey of the membership of the society. She found that only 17% of sufferers had received physiotherapy, 13% occupational therapy, and a mere 3% speech therapy. In addition, 54% had never spoken with a social worker, and 60% had never spoken with a health visitor, though 50% live with a spouse who is suffering from illness, and 17% live alone.

Using continual customer research and a client-centred approach, the Welfare Department's first priority is to respond to the individual's needs which may be emotional, medical, spiritual, financial, practical or a combination of these. Where there is hardship the society can sometimes make specific 'one-off' grants to help purchase special items such as wheelchairs, holidays, etc. The society endeavours to provide as much help as possible and seeks funding on the client's behalf from other sources such as benevolent funds and statutory sources for nursing home fees.

The Welfare Department also tries to build a bridge between the customer (both patients and carers) and the service providers (i.e. the power base of politicians, doctors and caring professionals). For instance our Welfare and Benefits Officer will lobby politicians about issues that arise from the queries that our clients bring to her about benefits, prescriptions, aids for the disabled, etc. the Education Officer through her study days targets the doctors and nurses who are responsible for the medical care of sufferers, as well as the therapists who maintain and improve their quality of life. In so doing it is hoped to foster awareness by these professionals of the special problems of PD.

The Regional Welfare Co-ordinators build up networks of local services to improve and sustain local resources and bring the needs of our clients to the attention of local statutory and voluntary bodies. The Welfare Department also supports a number of welfare-orientated research projects aimed at improving services and the quality of life for sufferers.

The welfare programme is guided by the society's Welfare Advisory Panel, which geographically and professionally have very wide and valuable experience to draw upon. The Panel considers any new project applications for welfare research as well as discussing any government policies which may have an effect on the society, matters of the society's policy relating to welfare issues, and generally any other aspects of welfare work that are referred to it.

The aim of these projects is to establish models of good practice to dovetail into the existing system. They may be concerned to help the sufferer and/or carer, or they may be concerned to improve services relating to a particular profession or area of therapeutic work. Many have a relevance to other neurological conditions, and where possible the involvement of other relevant charities is sought.

One of the most important projects set up by the Welfare Department has been the Neuro-care team Project. This had the aim of devising a model for the management of PD and putting it into practice within a NHS neurology department. This involved the establishment of a multidisciplinary neuro-care team, which also aimed to deal with other neurological conditions such as motor neurone disease, dystonia, Friedreich's ataxia, and multiple sclerosis. Other projects include studies of the needs of people with PD and their families with an emphasis on terminal care, of the role of the GP in the care of PD sufferers, and of a disability clinic. The latter aims to develop a model system for integrating the care of disabled people in the community. Another project is the development of a diary which the patient can use to keep records on all aspects of the disease and any other relevant factors such as the use of other medications.

In addition there are working parties in physiotherapy, speech therapy and nursing, all staffed by professionals active in the field; they have produced a wealth of information for use by their own professions. The physiotherapy and speech therapy working parties have helped to publicize the value of their expertise in helping PD patients. The nursing working party was formed in response to letters received from clients about their experiences when admitted to hospital. They have produced a poster for nurses, highlighting some of the most common problems associated with PD and are now working on an information pack to complement the poster. An occupational therapy working party will be set up in the near future; initial surveys about aids and equipment have already been carried out.

The Welfare Department recognizes the needs of the carer as being equally important to those of the sufferer, and much of their work has focused on the carer. A research team has been studying the psychosocial aspects of PD, with the emphasis on the impact on the carer. This research has produced some very interesting findings and the team are hoping to be able to extend this project in order to develop a treatment package which will include medical and emotional aspects as well as providing information and practical help for the carer. Allied to this is a project looking into the possibility of establishing small respite care units within hospitals where the patient and carer could be admitted together if appropriate. This would enable the carer to have a break without being separated from her partner, with the opportunity for assessment of both persons' needs and the existing services available to them. Extra services including physiotherapy and occupational therapy would be available, and the unit would be suitable not only for PD sufferers but other neurological conditions as well.

Much of our work with carers is done in co-operation with the Carers National Association, an organization specifically for carers, who provide speakers at seminars and study days which the society runs. We also have links with organizations such as Crossroads which provides respite care services.

Another important area of work involving respite care is the provision of holidays, either for a couple (with the care provided for the sufferer in order to relieve the carer) or for the sufferer alone. The Welfare Department run a series of special holidays every year in conjunction with the Winged Fellowship Trust as well as a holiday abroad. It also gives advice on individual requests for holidays and help locate sources of funding. In the past, therapy fortnights involving speech therapy, physiotherapy, art and music therapy, and yoga have been provided.

The society also supports the work of the foundation for Conductive Education in Birmingham, which has been set up, with some funding from the society, to provide in Britain, the revolutionary teaching system for people with physical disabilities developed at the Peto Institute in Hungary. Evaluation is still in process but many PD sufferers who have visited the Peto Institute have found it beneficial.

The needs of the younger sufferer are another important aspect of welfare work. PD is often misrepresented as 'an old person's disease', but the needs of both old and young are equally important. Those of the younger sufferer can be different from the older person. They are often juggling with family relationships, employment and financial constraints such as mortgages, in addition to PD. They often feel isolated by their age amongst other PD sufferers and their particular problems need to be addressed. As a result of requests, from this younger age group, the society has hosted a series of seminars. Information and speakers have been provided on many topics, the Welfare Department acting on the needs expressed by the participants. From a small beginning, the numbers of participants in these weekends has increased each year, as news of the weekends spread and more younger sufferers have been identified. The weekends have become a major way of identifying needs and trying to find a solution for some of the problems that these younger sufferers face.

The YAPP&RS (Young Alert Parkinsonians Partners and Relatives) were formed in April 1988. Their magazine is edited by a committee of sufferers. Their activites are growing steadily. They are a very valuable asset to the society and are often used as a resource at study days. It has to be said that their input based on personal experience has proved to be extremely valuable to the professionals attending the study days. Discussions on family relationships have led to a project in conjunction with the National Children's Bureau looking into the needs of children who have a parent with PD. Concerns about driving have led to a project to establish a driving centre for the disabled. A survey on sexual problems has been carried out; it is hoped that the findings will highlight areas of concern where help can be given.

The Welfare Department is now working on the possibility of establishing links with the churches to encourage their involvement in the pastoral care of PD sufferers. Another priority is to identify the needs of people from ethnic minority groups who suffer from PD, in the hope of providing appropriate support for them.

BRANCHES

There are currently 160 local branches of the society throughout the country. The character and activities of each branch vary enormously, but their main aim is to provide mutual self-help and support and the opportunity for a socal life, isolation being a common problem for people suffering from PD. Branch Development Officers are employed to act as midwives bringing branches into being and providing support afterwards. This is often a difficult birth, the branch being vulnerable to the vagaries of PD. Yet amazingly once born, they cling to life with great tenacity.

The work done by the branches in fund-raising and providing social activities for their members is considerable. In addition many engage in welfare work and provide an invaluable resource to the society's staff, particularly the Regional Welfare Co-ordinators and the Education Officer who often involves them in study days. Some of the branches have also set up their own initiatives. It is important that professionals recognize their worth and refer people to them for help as self-help groups such as these can make an important difference to the sufferer and carer's quality of life. They enable people to speak about and share their problems with others in similar situations. They can also deal with problems and act as a pressure group at a local level as well as disseminating information and working together to improve conditions for those who have PD. The society could not do without their strength and wisdom.

To provide support for the branches, the society runs a series of weekend seminars for representatives of branches. All parts of the society contribute to these seminars, which provide an invaluable opportunity for the branches to meet each other and exchange ideas.

CONCLUSION

It is hoped that the work currently done in all areas of the society will continue to grow and that the work that Mali Jenkins started in 1969 will continue to flourish to the benefit of Parkinson's disease sufferers and their families.

REFERENCES

Banks, M.A. and Caird, F.I. (1989) Physiotherapy benefits patients with Parkinson's disease. *Clinical Rehabilitation*, **3**, 11–16.

Lees, A.J. (1988) Brain Tissue Bank. *Parkinson's Disease Society Newsletter,* **65**, 23–4.

Oxtoby, M. (1982) *Parkinson's Disease Patients and their Social Needs.* Parkinson's Disease Society, London, 14, 29, and 32.

Pearce, V. (1989) Notes on Apomorphine (unpublished).

Strange, P. (1989) The Lock which Fits the Key – Isolation of the Receptor for Dopamine in the Brain. *Parkinson's Disease Society Newsletter,* **68**, 5.

Truscott, T.G. (1988) Chemically-induced Parkinson's disease. *Parkinson's Disease Society Newsletter,* **66**, 16.

Useful addresses

Age Concern England

60 Pitcairn Road
Mitcham
Surrey
CR4 3LL
Tel: 081 640 5431

British Red Cross Society

9 Grosvenor Crescent
Mitcham
London
SW1X 7EJ
Tel: 071 235 5454

Counsel & Care for the Elderly

Twyman House
16 Bonny Street
London
NW1 9LR
Tel: 071 485 1566

Carers National Association

29 Chilworth Mews
London
W2 3RG
Tel: 071 724 7776

Carematch

286 Camden Road
London
N7 0BJ
Tel: 071 609 9966

Crossroads Care Attendant Scheme

10 Regent Place
Rugby
Warwickshire
CV21 2PN
Tel: 0788 72653

Cruse, Bereavement Care

126 Sheen Road
Richmond
TW9 1UR
Tel: 081 940 4818

DIAL UK

177 High Street
Clay Cross
Chesterfield
Derbyshire
S45 9DZ
Tel: 0246 25055

Disability Alliance	25 Denmark Street London WC2 8NJ Tel: 071 240 0846
Disabled Living Foundation	380–384 Harrow Road London W9 2HU Tel: 071 289 6111
Elderly Accommodation Counsel	31 Kensington Court London W8 5BH Tel: 071 937 8709
Gardens for the Disabled Trust	Membership Secretary Church Cottage Headcorn Kent TN27 9NP
Holiday Care Service	2 Old Bank Chambers Station Road Horley Surrey RH6 9HW
Horticultural Therapy	Goulds Ground Vallis Way Frome Somerset BA11 3DW Tel: 0373 64782
Royal Association for Disability Rehabilitation (RADAR)	25 Mortimer Street London W1N 8AB Tel: 071 637 5400
Scottish Council on Disability/Disability Scotland	Princes House 5 Shandwick Place Edinburgh EH2 4RG Tel: 031 229 8632
SPOD (The Association to Aid the Sexual and Personal Relationships of People with a Disability)	286 Camden Road London N7 0BJ Tel: 071 607 8851

Tripscope – Transport Information for People with Disabilities

63 Esmond Road
London
W4 1JE
Tel: 081 994 9294

Wales Council for the Disabled

Llys Ifor
Crescent Road
Caerphilly
Mid Glamorgan
CF8 1XL
Tel: 0222 887325

Winged Fellowship Trust

Holidays for the Disabled
Angel House
Pentonville Road
London
N1 9XD
Tel: 071 833 2594

Index

Accidents 28
Acetylcholine 9
Agitation 10, 13
Akathisia 11, 22
Akinesia 17
Alcohol 32
Allowances 115
Alzheimer's disease 1, 13
Amantadine 9, 13, 15
Anaesthesia 42
Analgesia 19, 39
Analyser
  computerized voice 94
  glottal frequency 94
Anorexia 10, 31
Anticholiergic 8, 9, 13, 14, 33
Antidepressant 19
Antiemetic 10
Anxiety 10, 19, 32, 38, 40, 57
Anxiolytic 19
Appetite 10
Artane 9
Articulation 90
Assessment
  nursing 25
  physiotherapy 46
  speech therapy 94
  swallowing 99
Aspiration 31
Autonomic failure, progressive 1

Bath 78
  rail 79
  seat 79
Bathing 34, 108
Bed 28, 76
  blocks 76
  cage 76
  clothes 39
Belladona 8
Benefits 115
Benzhexol 9, 13
Benztropine 9, 13
Blinking 4
Bradykinesia 4, 23, 38, 47, 66
Brain bank 119
Breathing exercises 30, 57
Bromocriptine 9, 12, 15–7
Bulking agents 33

Caffeine 32
Can-opener 83
Cannabis 8
Cardiac arrhythmias 10, 12
Carers 42, 51, 71, 93, 113, 116–8
Caudate nucleus 3, 21
Chair 28, 36, 56, 74
Cholinergic 9, 13
Chorea 11
Choreoathetosis 11
Cigarette smoking 2
Clothing 28, 78

Cogentin 9
Communication 68, 108, 115
  board 96
Community
  nurse 42, 43, 114
  occupational therapist 70
Compliance 19, 61, 62
Conductive education 54, 124
Constipation 14, 19, 32, 33
Continence nurse 114
Cooking 83
Cough 31
Crafts 69
Crockery 31, 84
Cryosurgery 20
Cutlery 31, 84, 101

DAF 95
Decarboxylase inhibitor 9
Delusions 10, 14, 21
Dementia 5, 6, 13, 19, 30, 41
Dental care 114
Denture 101
Deprenyl 9
Depression 5, 10, 19, 21, 30, 31,
    38, 40, 55, 90, 108
Diclofenac 19
Disipal 9
Domiciliary physiotherapy 63
Domperidone 10
Dopamine 3
Dopaminergic 15, 19
Dorsal vagal nuclei 9
Dosette 19
Dressing 34, 77, 108
  aids 78
Drooling 39, 87, 101
Drowsiness 14
Drug holiday 18
Dry mouth 14, 21, 32, 99
Dycem mat 76, 83, 84
Dysarthria 22, 87, 88
  therapy 98
Dyskinesia 10–13, 16, 17, 28, 40
  orofacial, orolingual 11, 22, 92

Dysphagia 99
Dysprosody 88
Dystonia 11, 40

Elastic stocking 28
Eldepryl 9
Electroconvulsive therapy 8
Erythromelalgia 12
Eye movements 5

Face 4, 5, 23, 30, 95
Faecal softeners 33
Fatigue 71
Feeding 83
Festination 4, 28
Footwear 28
Freezing 5, 28, 35, 38, 40, 58, 115

Gait 22, 23, 35, 48–9, 58
Gardening 72
Glaucoma 13
Glottal frequency analysers 94
Goniometry 49
Grab rail 79, 80

Hallucinations 5, 10, 14, 21, 40, 41
Hand rail 33, 39, 74
Handwriting 23
Head injury 1
Helping hand 74
Hemlock 8
Hobbies 37, 72, 108
Holidays 116, 120, 124
Hydrotherapy 54, 97
Hypokinesia 4, 14, 18
Hypothermia 34

Ibuprofen 19
Ice 95, 96, 101
Immobility 19, 34, 35, 39
Implants
  adrenal 20, 21
  foetal neural 20, 21
Incontinence 33
Infarction, cerebral 1

Intonation 88

Kitchen 81

Levodopa 8–10, 15, 33, 40, 45, 92
Levodopa-PDI 15–17, 23
Lewy bodies 3
Lifting 36, 37
Lisuride 12
Litewriter 96
Livedo reticularis 13
Locus coeruleus 9

Madopar 9, 10, 15, 16, 18
Meals-on-wheels 114
Meter, sound level 94
Metoclopramide 10
Mobility 22, 108, 109
Monoamine oxidase inhibitor 12
MPTP 1, 2, 12, 23, 119
Multiple system atrophy 1
Music therapy 96

Nausea 10
Nightmares 40
NSAI 19
Nursing home 118

Obesity 32
Occupational therapist 66, 114
Oedema 13
Olivopontocerebellar atrophy 1
On–off phenomenon 5, 17, 22, 35, 71, 115
Opium 8
Orphenadrine 9, 13
Osteoarthrosis 19

Pain 113
Pallidectomy 20
Paracetamol 19
Paranoid state 10, 14, 21
Parkinson's disease, Parkinsonism
  prevalence 2
  sex incidence 2
    post-encephalitic 1
    idiopathic 1, 3
    drug induced 1
Parlodel 9
PDI 10
PDS (Parkinson's Disease
  Society) 98, 102, 110, 115–9
Pergolide 12
Phonation 90
Picture board 30
PNF 52
Posture, postural 45, 48
  hypotension 10, 12, 28
  instability 4
  reflexes 18
Pressure sores 35
Prosodic therapy 95
Prosody 88, 92
Prostatism 14, 19
Purgative 19

Rating scale 22, 23
Residential care 118
Respiration 89, 96
Respite care 118
Restlessness 13, 14
Retention 14
Rigidity 4, 18, 19, 23, 38, 47, 57, 66, 87
Rope ladder 39

Salivation 5
Scalding 28
Seborrhoea 5, 23
Selegiline 9, 15–17
Sex 38, 39
Shaving 80
Sheltered accommodation 118
Shopping 83
Shower 79, 80
Shy–Drager syndrome 1
Sinemet 9, 10, 15, 16
Sitting 56
  posture 28
Sleep 39, 40
Speech 5, 23

amplification 97
therapist 21, 29, 68
Spinal rotation 47
Standing 4, 36
Steele–Richardson syndrome 1
Stereotactic surgery 20
Stramonium 8
Strionigral degeneration 1
Substantia nigra 3, 9
Supranuclear palsy, progressive 1
Surgical treatment 19, 20,
Swallowing 5, 30, 31, 84, 98
Symmetrel 9

Telephone 74
Thalamotomy 20
Toilet 28, 80, 113
seat 33

Tremor 4, 15, 18, 23, 38, 46, 57, 66, 83
essential 6
senile 6
Trolley 81, 82
Turning 4

Vasospasm, digital 12
Velcro 78
Videofluoroscopy 100

Walking 14, 35, 108
aid 28, 59
Walkway 49
Washing 34
Wearing-off 17
Wheelchair 60, 120
Writing 23, 69

YAPP&RS 125